I0706707

UNDERSTANDING TYPE 2 DIABETES

Simple guide to reduce blood sugar, medical expenses,and stay healthy always.

Copyright © 2024 by [ANGEL MORAN]

All rights reserved. No part of this publication may be reproduced, distributed, or transmitted in any form or by any means, including photocopying, recording, or other electronic or mechanical methods, without the prior written permission of the publisher, except in the case of brief quotations embodied in critical reviews and certain other noncommercial uses permitted by copyright law.

Table of contents

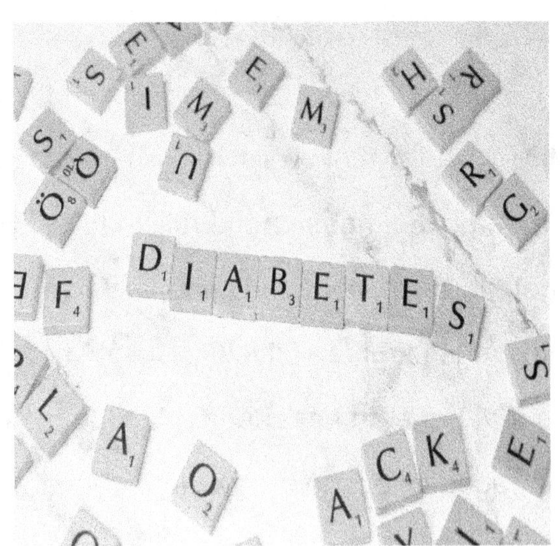

INTRODUCTION

In the quiet town of Wellsville, where the sun painted golden hues on the rolling hills, lived Angel Moran, a vibrant woman known for her infectious laughter. Little did the townsfolk know that beneath her cheerful facade, a silent battle raged within her body. Angel Moran was grappling with Type 2 diabetes, a condition that silently tiptoed into her life.

As we delve into the intricacies of Understanding Type 2 Diabetes, we follow Angel journey – a journey that mirrors the experiences of millions around the world. It's a story of resilience, adaptation, and the quest for knowledge in the face of a formidable aadversary.Angel initial confusion and fear morphed into a relentless pursuit of understanding. She sought guidance from healthcare professionals, delved into research, and connected with a supportive community. The story unfolds against a backdrop of changing lifestyles, where dietary habits and sedentary routines intertwine with genetic predispositions, leading to a rising tide of Type 2 diabetes diagnoses.

The narrative isn't just Angel; it intertwines with the broader tapestry of society grappling with a health crisis. We explore the factors contributing to the surge in Type 2 diabetes cases, demystifying the science behind the condition. From insulin resistance to blood sugar management, each chapter illuminates a piece of the puzzle.

Understanding Type 2 Diabetes becomes a beacon of knowledge, shedding light on prevention, management, and the role of a supportive community in the face of this prevalent health challenge. In Wellsville and beyond, Angel Moran story unfolds not as an isolated incident but as a microcosm of a global health concern that demands our attention and understanding.

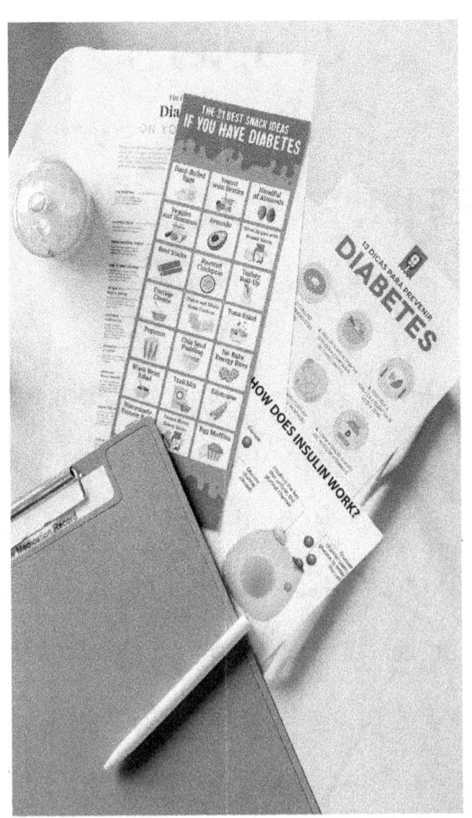
THE 21 BEST SNACK IDEAS
IF YOU HAVE DIABETES
13 DICAS PARA PREVENIR
DIABETES
HOW DOES INSULIN WORK?

Chapter 1

DEFINITION OF TYPE 2 DIABETES

Type 2 diabetes is a chronic metabolic disorder characterized by insulin resistance and impaired insulin secretion, leading to elevated blood glucose levels. Insulin, a hormone produced by the pancreas, normally facilitates the uptake of glucose by cells for energy. In individuals with type 2 diabetes, cells become resistant to insulin's actions, and the pancreas struggles to produce enough insulin.

Risk factors for type 2 diabetes include genetics, obesity, sedentary lifestyle, and age. The condition often develops gradually, and early stages may go unnoticed. Symptoms can

Prevalence and impact of type 2 diabetes

According to the World Health Organization (WHO), the number of people with diabetes rose from 108 million in 1980 to 422 million in 2014.Compared to high-income countries, the prevalence of Type 2 diabetes has been increasing more quickly in low- and middle-income nations.Diabetes is a leading cause of lower limb amputation, heart attacks, strokes, blindness, and renal failure.. In 2019, diabetes and kidney disease due to diabetes caused an estimated 2 million deaths.A normal body weight, regular exercise, a balanced diet, and quitting smoking are all strategies to stop or prevent the development of type 2 diabetes.

The International Diabetes Federation (IDF) reports that 10.5% of the adult population

(20-79 years) has diabetes, with almost half unaware that they are living with the condition. By 2045, IDF projections show that 1 in 8 adults, approximately 783 million, will be living with diabetes, an increase of 46%. Over 90% of people with diabetes have type 2 diabetes, which is driven by socio-economic, demographic, environmental, and genetic factors.

Among the main causes of the increase of type 2 diabetes are:

- Urbanisation
- An ageing population
- Decreasing levels of physical activity
- Increasing overweight and obesity prevalence

On the other hand, diabetes can be lessened in severity by preventing diabetes with type 2 and treating all forms of the disease with appropriate treatment and an early diagnosis. Those who are living with the illness can prevent or avoid difficulties by taking these steps.

A study published in the Journal of Epidemiology and Global Health estimated that in 2017, approximately 462 million individuals were affected by type 2 diabetes corresponding to 6.28% of the world's population (4.4% of those aged 15–49 years, 15% of those aged 50–69, and 22% of those aged 70+), or a prevalence rate of 6059 cases per 100,000. The study also projected that by 2030, the number of people with type 2 diabetes will increase to 578 million (7.02% of the world's population), and by 2045, to 700 million (7.63% of the world's population). The study highlighted the need for more effective prevention and management strategies to reduce the burden of type 2 diabetes globally.

Type 2 diabetes is a serious and growing health problem that affects millions of people worldwide. It has significant social, economic, and human costs. By understanding the prevalence and impact of type 2 diabetes, we can take action to prevent, treat, and control this condition.

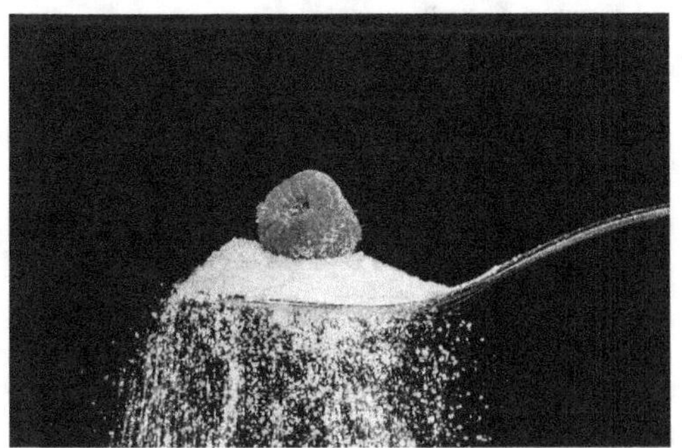

CHAPTER 2

CAUSES AND RISK FACTORS

Type 2 diabetes is a chronic condition that affects how the body regulates and uses glucose (sugar) as a fuel. People with type 2 diabetes either do not produce enough insulin, a hormone that helps cells take in glucose, or are resistant to the effects of insulin, meaning that their cells do not respond well to it. As a result, glucose builds up in the blood and can cause serious health problems over time.

Some of the causes and risk factors for developing type 2 diabetes are:

- **Weight.** Being overweight or obese increases the risk of type 2 diabetes, especially if the excess fat is stored around the abdomen. This is because abdominal fat can interfere with the action of insulin and make the body more resistant to it[12].

- **Age.** The risk of type 2 diabetes increases with age, as the body becomes less sensitive to insulin and the pancreas produces less of it. Although type 2 diabetes can occur at any age, it is more common in people older than 35 years.
- **Family history.** Having a parent, sibling, or other close relative with type 2 diabetes increases the likelihood of developing the condition, as it may indicate a genetic predisposition or shared environmental factors.
- **Race and ethnicity.** Some racial and ethnic groups have a higher risk of type 2 diabetes than others, such as African Americans, American Indians, Asian Americans, Hispanics/Latinos, and Pacific Islanders. This may be due to genetic, cultural, or socioeconomic factors that affect the prevalence of obesity, physical activity, diet, and access to health care.
- **Physical activity.** Being physically inactive reduces the body's ability to use

glucose and increases the risk of type 2 diabetes. Regular physical activity can help lower blood glucose levels, improve insulin sensitivity, and prevent weight gain.

- **Diet.** Eating a poor diet that is high in calories, fat, sugar, and refined carbohydrates can contribute to weight gain, insulin resistance, and type 2 diabetes. A healthy diet that is rich in fiber, protein, and complex carbohydrates can help prevent or manage type 2 diabetes.
- **Prediabetes.** Prediabetes is a condition where blood glucose levels are higher than normal, but not high enough to be diagnosed as diabetes. People with prediabetes have a higher risk of developing type 2 diabetes within 10 years, unless they make lifestyle changes to lower their blood glucose levels.
- **Gestational diabetes.**Diabetes that occurs during pregnancy, usually across either the second or third trimester, is known as gestational diabetes. . It affects both the mother and the baby, and increases the risk of complications such as high blood pressure, preterm

delivery, and birth defects. Women who have had gestational diabetes or given birth to a baby weighing more than 9 pounds are more likely to develop type 2 diabetes later in life.

- **Other health conditions.** Some health conditions can increase the risk of type 2 diabetes, such as polycystic ovary syndrome (PCOS), a hormonal disorder that affects women of reproductive age; Cushing's syndrome, a condition that causes excess cortisol production; and acromegaly, a condition that causes excess growth hormone production. These conditions can affect the body's metabolism and insulin secretion.
- **Medications.** Some medications can affect blood glucose levels and increase the risk of type 2 diabetes, such as steroids, antipsychotics, and HIV drugs. These medications should be used with caution and under medical supervision, and their effects on blood glucose should be monitored regularly.

GENETICS

Genetics is a branch of biology that studies how traits are inherited and passed on from one generation to the next. It involves the structure and function of genes, chromosomes, and DNA, as well as the interactions between them and the environment. Genetics can help explain why some people are more likely to develop certain diseases, such as type 2 diabetes, than others.

Some of the main topics in genetics are:

- **Mendelian genetics**: This is the study of how traits are inherited according to the laws of segregation and independent assortment, discovered by

Gregor Mendel in the 19th century. Mendel used pea plants to demonstrate that traits are controlled by discrete units of inheritance, now known as genes, and that each parent contributes one copy of each gene to the offspring. Mendelian genetics also explains how traits can be dominant or recessive, and how they can be influenced by the sex of the individual.

- **Molecular genetics**: This is the study of the molecular structure and function of genes and their products, such as proteins and RNA. Molecular genetics reveals how genes are encoded in DNA, how they are transcribed into RNA, and how they are translated into proteins. Molecular genetics also explores how genes are regulated, how they can mutate, and how they can be manipulated using techniques such as gene cloning, gene editing, and gene therapy.

- **Population genetics**: This is the study of the genetic variation and evolution of populations of organisms. Population genetics examines how gene frequencies change over time due to factors such as natural selection, genetic drift, gene flow, and mutation. Population genetics also analyzes how genetic diversity affects the adaptation, speciation, and extinction of species.

- **Genomics**: This is the study of the complete set of genes and their interactions in an organism or a group of organisms. Genomics uses technologies such as DNA sequencing, bioinformatics, and comparative genomics to map, analyze, and compare the genomes of different organisms. Genomics can reveal the origin, function, and evolution of genes, as well as their role in health and disease.

LIFESTYLE FACTORS

Lifestyle factors are the habits, behaviors, and attitudes that influence the health and well-being of individuals and populations. Lifestyle factors can have positive or negative effects on physical, mental, and social health. Some examples of lifestyle factors are:

.Diet: The food and drinks that people consume can affect their weight, nutrition, digestion, immunity, and risk of various diseases.For optimum health, a balanced diet rich in whole grains, lean meats, fruits, vegetables, and healthy fats is advised. A poor diet that is high in processed foods, sugar, salt, and saturated fats can lead to obesity, diabetes, heart disease, and some cancers

.Physical activity: The amount and type of exercise that people do can influence their fitness, strength, endurance, flexibility, and mood. Physical activity can also prevent or manage many chronic conditions, such as hypertension, cardiovascular disease, diabetes, osteoporosis, and depression.

- **Sleep**: The quality and quantity of sleep that people get can affect their energy, concentration, memory, mood, and immune system. Sleep also plays a role in regulating hormones, metabolism, and inflammation. Lack of sleep or poor sleep quality can increase the risk of obesity, diabetes, cardiovascular disease, and mental disorders. The National Sleep Foundation recommends that adults get seven to nine hours of sleep per night, and that they follow good sleep hygiene practices, such as having a regular bedtime routine, avoiding caffeine and alcohol before bed, and minimizing light and noise in the bedroom .

- **Smoking**: Smoking tobacco products is one of the most harmful lifestyle factors, as it causes damage to nearly every organ in the body and increases the risk of many diseases, such as lung cancer, chronic obstructive pulmonary disease (COPD), stroke, and coronary heart disease. Smoking also affects the health of non-smokers who are exposed to secondhand smoke. Quitting smoking can reduce the risk of these diseases and improve the quality of life. There are various methods and resources available to help smokers quit, such as nicotine replacement therapy, counseling, and support groups .

.Alcohol consumption: Drinking alcohol can have both positive and negative effects on health, depending on the amount and frequency of consumption. Moderate alcohol consumption, defined as up to one drink per day for women and up to two drinks per day for men, may have some protective effects against cardiovascular disease and diabetes. However, excessive alcohol consumption, defined as more than four drinks per day for men and more than three drinks per day for women, can increase the risk of liver disease, pancreatitis, cancer, and mental disorders. Alcohol can also impair judgment, coordination, and reaction time, and increase the likelihood of accidents, injuries, and violence. Therefore, it is important to drink responsibly and limit alcohol intake to the recommended levels

These are some of the main lifestyle factors that can affect health and longevity. By making positive changes in these areas, people can improve their health outcomes and quality of life. However, lifestyle factors are not the only determinants of health. There are also other factors, such as genetics, environment, socioeconomic status, and health care access, that can influence health and well-being. Therefore, it is important to consider the whole picture of health and address the multiple factors that contribute to it.

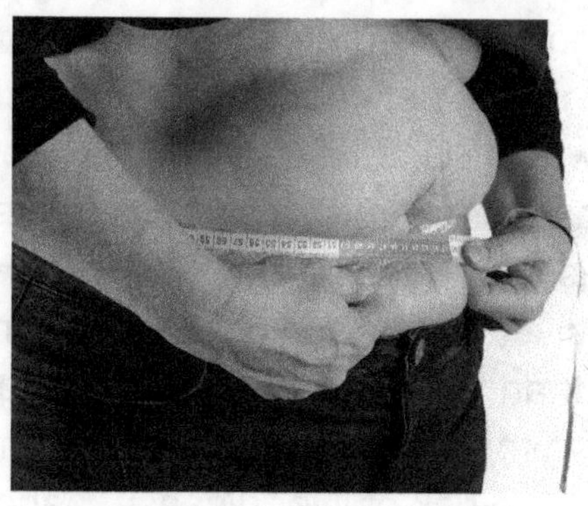

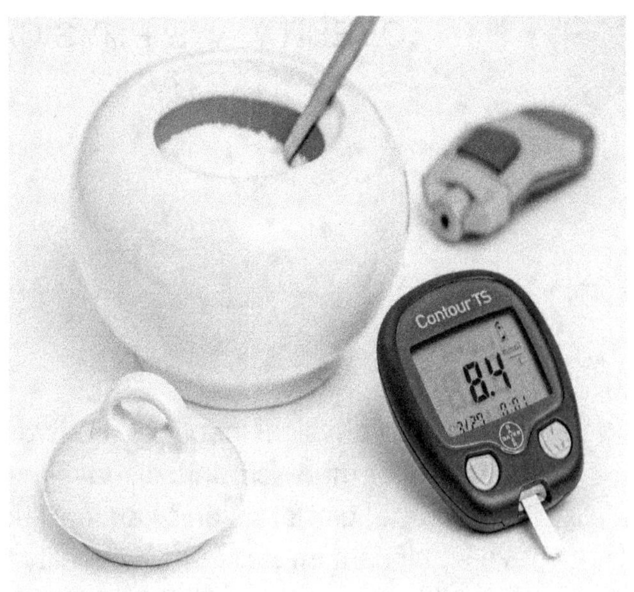

OBESITY AND PHYSICAL INACTIVITY

Obesity and physical inactivity are two major risk factors for many chronic diseases, such as heart disease, diabetes, and cancer. They also have significant impacts on the quality of life, health care costs, and productivity of individuals and populations. In this essay, I will discuss the causes, consequences, and prevention strategies of obesity and physical inactivity, using evidence from web search results. A body mass index, or BMI of 30 or greater, which denotes extra body fat, is considered obese. Physical inactivity is defined as not meeting the recommended levels of moderate-to-vigorous physical activity, which are at least 150 minutes per week for adults and 60 minutes per day for children. Both obesity and physical inactivity can result from a complex interplay of genetic, biological, behavioral, environmental, and social factors. Some of the common causes include:

- **Energy imbalance**: Consuming more calories than burning through physical activity leads to weight gain and obesity. Many people today have easy access to high-calorie, low-nutrient foods and beverages, while facing barriers to physical activity, such as lack of time, facilities, safety, or motivation.
- **Sedentary lifestyle**: Spending more time on screen-based activities, such as watching TV, playing video games, or using computers, reduces the time and opportunity for physical activity. Sedentary behaviors can also disrupt the normal patterns of appetite and metabolism, leading to overeating and weight gain.
- **Genetic predisposition**: Some people may have inherited genes that make them more prone to obesity or less responsive to physical activity. For example, some gene variants can affect the regulation of hunger, satiety, fat storage, or energy expenditure. However, genes alone cannot explain the rapid rise of obesity and physical inactivity in recent decades, as the genetic makeup of populations has not changed significantly in that period.

Obesity and physical inactivity can have serious health consequences, both individually and synergistically. Some of the major health problems associated with obesity and physical inactivity are:

- **Cardiovascular disease**: Excess body fat, especially around the waist, can increase the risk of high blood pressure, high cholesterol, and inflammation, which can damage the blood vessels and the heart. Physical inactivity can also weaken the heart muscle and reduce its efficiency. Together, obesity and physical inactivity can lead to coronary heart disease, stroke, heart failure, and other complications.
- **Type 2 diabetes**: Obesity can impair the body's ability to use insulin, the hormone that regulates blood sugar levels. Physical inactivity can also reduce the sensitivity of the cells to insulin, resulting in high blood sugar levels. Over time, this can cause type 2 diabetes, which can damage the eyes, kidneys, nerves, and other organs.
- **Cancer**: Obesity can alter the levels of hormones, such as estrogen, testosterone, and insulin, which can

affect the growth and division of cells. Physical inactivity can also reduce the immune system's ability to fight off infections and abnormal cells. Together, obesity and physical inactivity can increase the risk of cancers of the breast, colon, uterus, and other sites.

- **Mental health**: Obesity can affect the self-esteem, body image, and mood of individuals, leading to depression, anxiety, and social isolation. Physical inactivity can also reduce the production of endorphins, the natural chemicals that enhance the mood and relieve stress. Together, obesity and physical inactivity can impair the mental health and well-being of individuals.

Obesity and physical inactivity are preventable and treatable conditions, and there are many effective strategies to address them. Some of the key strategies include:

- **Dietary modification**: Reducing the intake of calories, especially from added sugars, saturated fats, and refined grains, and increasing the intake of fruits, vegetables, whole grains, lean proteins, and healthy fats, can help achieve and maintain a healthy weight and prevent obesity. Eating a balanced and varied diet can also provide the essential nutrients and antioxidants that support the health and function of the body.

- **Physical activity promotion**: Increasing the frequency, intensity, duration, and variety of physical activity, both aerobic and muscle-strengthening, can help burn calories, improve fitness, and prevent physical inactivity. Engaging in physical activity can also provide many benefits, such as improving the mood, sleep quality, cognitive ability, bone and musculoskeletal health, and immune system.
- **Environmental and policy changes**: Creating and enhancing the physical and social environments that support and encourage physical activity and healthy eating, such as providing safe and accessible parks, trails, sidewalks, bike lanes, playgrounds, schools, workplaces, and communities, can help overcome the barriers and challenges that people face in their daily lives. Implementing and enforcing policies that regulate the availability, affordability, and marketing of healthy and unhealthy

foods and beverages, such as taxes, subsidies, labels, and bans, can also help influence the choices and behaviors of individuals and populations.

In conclusion, obesity and physical inactivity are major public health problems that affect millions of people worldwide. They are caused by a complex interaction of multiple factors, and they can lead to many chronic diseases and reduced quality of life. However, they are also preventable and treatable, and there are many effective strategies to address them. By adopting a healthy lifestyle, creating a supportive environment, and implementing sound policies, we can reduce the burden of obesity and physical inactivity and improve the health and well-being of ourselves and others.

CHAPTER 3

PATHOPHYSIOLOGY

underlying processes and interactions that lead to them. Pathophysiology can also provide the basis for developing diagnostic tests, treatments, and preventive measures for various diseases.

Some examples of pathophysiology are:

- Diabetes mellitus: a chronic metabolic disorder characterized by hyperglycemia (high blood sugar) due to insufficient insulin production or action. Diabetes can cause various complications, such as cardiovascular disease, kidney failure, nerve damage, and eye problems. The pathophysiology of diabetes involves the impairment of glucose uptake and utilization by cells, the accumulation of glucose and other substances in the blood and tissues, and the activation of inflammatory and oxidative stress pathways.
- Asthma: a chronic inflammatory disorder of the airways that causes wheezing,

coughing, chest tightness, and shortness of breath. Asthma can be triggered by allergens, infections, exercise, stress, or other factors. The pathophysiology of asthma involves the hypersensitivity of the immune system to certain stimuli, the constriction and inflammation of the bronchial tubes, the increased mucus production and secretion, and the remodeling of the airway structure and function.

- Alzheimer's disease: a progressive neurodegenerative disorder that causes memory loss, cognitive decline, and behavioral changes. The most typical root cause of dementia in older persons is Alzheimer's disease. The pathophysiology of Alzheimer's disease involves the accumulation of amyloid-beta plaques and neurofibrillary tangles in the brain, the loss of synapses and neurons, the disruption of neurotransmission and signaling, and the activation of neuroinflammation and oxidative stress pathways.

These are just some of the many examples of pathophysiology that can help us to understand the nature and progression of diseases, as well as to find ways to diagnose, treat, and prevent them. Pathophysiology is a complex and dynamic field that requires interdisciplinary collaboration and integration of knowledge from various disciplines, such as anatomy, physiology, biochemistry, genetics, immunology, microbiology, pharmacology, and epidemiology. Pathophysiology is also an essential component of medical education and practice.

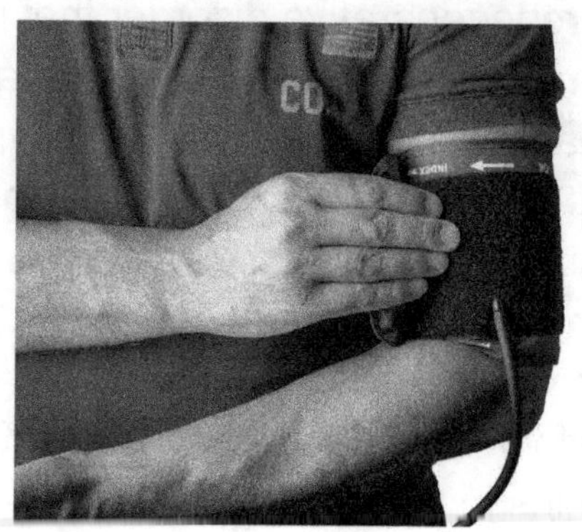

INSULLIN RESISTANCE

Insulin resistance is a condition in which the body does not respond properly to the hormone insulin, which helps regulate blood sugar levels. Insulin resistance can lead to high blood sugar levels, which can cause various health problems, such as prediabetes, Type 2 diabetes, obesity, cardiovascular disease, nonalcoholic fatty liver disease, and polycystic ovary syndrome.

Some of the possible causes of insulin resistance are:

- Obesity, especially excess fat around the waist
- Lack of physical activity
- High intake of carbohydrates
- Family history of diabetes
- Ethnicity (African, Latino, and Native American are at higher risk)
- Hormonal disorders, such as Cushing's syndrome and acromegaly
- Medications, such as steroids, antipsychotics, and HIV drugs
- Sleep problems, such as sleep apnea
- Stress
- Infection or illness

Insulin resistance does not have any specific symptoms until it leads to high blood sugar levels. Some of the signs of high blood sugar levels are:

- Frequent urination
- Excessive thirst
- Hunger
- Fatigue
- Blurred vision
- Darkening of the skin in the armpits, neck, and groin
- Irregular periods in women

Insulin resistance can be diagnosed by a doctor through a physical exam and blood tests, such as:

- Fasting plasma glucose test, which measures blood sugar after fasting for at least 8 hours
- Oral glucose tolerance test, which measures blood sugar before and 2 hours after drinking a sugary solution
- Hemoglobin A1c test, which measures the average blood sugar level over the past 2 to 3 months
- Insulin level test, which measures the amount of insulin in the blood

One can prevent and cure insulin resistance by:

- Losing weight and maintaining a healthy weight
- Increasing physical activity and exercising regularly
- Consuming a diet rich in nutrients such as fiber, protein, and healthy fats and low in carbs
- Avoiding smoking and alcohol
- Managing stress and getting enough sleep
- Taking medications, such as metformin and pioglitazone, that can improve insulin sensitivity
- Monitoring blood sugar levels and taking insulin injections if needed

Insulin resistance is a serious condition that can have long-term complications, such as:

- Type 2 diabetes, which is a chronic disease that affects how the body uses glucose
- Cardiovascular disease, which is a group of diseases that affect the heart and blood vessels, such as heart attack and stroke

- Nonalcoholic fatty liver disease, which is a condition in which fat builds up in the liver and causes inflammation and scarring
- Metabolic syndrome, which is a cluster of risk factors for cardiovascular disease and diabetes, such as high blood pressure, high cholesterol, and high triglycerides
- Polycystic ovary syndrome, which is a hormonal disorder that affects women's reproductive health and can cause infertility, irregular periods, acne, and excess hair growth

Insulin resistance is a common and preventable condition that can be managed with lifestyle changes and medical care. By following the advice of your doctor and taking care of your health, you can reduce your risk of developing insulin resistance and its complications.

BETA-CELL DYSFUNCTION

Beta-cell dysfunction is a term that describes the impairment of insulin secretion by the pancreatic beta-cells, which are responsible for producing and releasing insulin in response to glucose and other stimuli. Beta-cell dysfunction is a key feature of type 2 diabetes, as it leads to chronic hyperglycemia and metabolic complications.

There are different factors that can contribute to beta-cell dysfunction, such as genetic predisposition, environmental triggers, oxidative stress, inflammation, lipotoxicity, glucotoxicity, amyloid deposition, and endoplasmic reticulum stress. These factors can affect the beta-cell mass, phenotype, and function in various ways, resulting in reduced insulin synthesis, secretion, and action.

Beta-cell dysfunction can be classified into five stages, according to the degree of glucose intolerance and the changes in beta-cell characteristics. These stages are:

- Stage 1: Compensation.At this point, insulin secretion rises to preserve glucose levels in the face of declining beta-cell mass and/or insulin resistance . The beta-cells retain their differentiated function and acute glucose-stimulated insulin secretion (GSIS).
- Stage 2: Adaptation. In this stage, glucose levels start to rise, reaching the range of impaired fasting glucose (IFG)

or impaired glucose tolerance (IGT). The beta-cells lose some of their mass and function, as evidenced by diminished GSIS and beta-cell dedifferentiation.

- Stage 3: Early decompensation. In this stage, glucose levels rise rapidly to the level of frank diabetes. The beta-cells undergo further dedifferentiation and loss of function, as well as increased apoptosis and senescence.
- Stage 4: Stable decompensation. In this stage, glucose levels remain high and stable, and the beta-cells show more severe dedifferentiation and dysfunction. The beta-cells may also exhibit altered morphology and gene expression, as well as increased oxidative stress and inflammation.
- Stage 5: Severe decompensation. In this stage, glucose levels become very high and unstable, and the beta-cells show a profound reduction in mass and function. The beta-cells may also develop insulin resistance and produce proinsulin instead of insulin. This stage is associated with the risk of ketoacidosis and diabetic complications.

The progression of beta-cell dysfunction can be influenced by various factors, such as the duration and severity of hyperglycemia, the degree of insulin resistance, the presence of autoimmunity, and the availability of therapeutic interventions. Some of the beta-cell dysfunction may be reversible, especially in the early stages, if the underlying causes are addressed and the metabolic stress is relieved. For example, weight loss, exercise, diet, and pharmacological agents can improve beta-cell function and glucose control in some patients with type 2 diabetes. However, in the later stages, the beta-cell dysfunction may become irreversible and require exogenous insulin replacement.

To summarize, beta-cell dysfunction is a complex and dynamic process that involves multiple mechanisms and stages. It is a major cause of type 2 diabetes and its complications. Understanding the pathophysiology and progression of beta-cell dysfunction can help in the prevention, diagnosis, and treatment of type 2 diabetes

GLUCOSE METABOLISM

Type 2 diabetes is a metabolic disorder that affects the body's ability to use glucose as a source of energy. Glucose is the main fuel for cells, and it comes from the food we eat, especially carbohydrates. Normally, when glucose enters the bloodstream, the pancreas releases insulin, a hormone that helps glucose move into cells. However, in type 2 diabetes, the body becomes resistant to insulin, meaning that it does not respond as well to the hormone.Consequently, the accumulation of glucose in the blood leads to elevated blood sugar levels.. This can lead to various complications, such as nerve damage, kidney damage, eye problems, and cardiovascular disease.

Glucose metabolism is the process of breaking down glucose and using it for energy or storing it for later use. There are three main pathways of glucose metabolism: glycolysis, gluconeogenesis, and glycogenolysis.

- Glycolysis is the breakdown of glucose into pyruvate, which can then be used for energy production in the mitochondria (the powerhouses of the cell) or converted into lactate. Glycolysis occurs in the cytoplasm (the fluid inside the cell) and does not require oxygen. It produces a small amount of ATP (the energy currency of the cell) and NADH (a molecule that carries electrons).
- Gluconeogenesis is the synthesis of glucose from non-carbohydrate sources, such as amino acids, lactate, glycerol, and pyruvate. Gluconeogenesis occurs mainly in the liver and kidneys, and it requires energy and oxygen. It helps maintain blood glucose levels during fasting, starvation, or intense exercise.

- Glycogenolysis is the breakdown of glycogen, a large molecule that stores glucose in the liver and muscles. Glycogenolysis releases glucose into the blood when it is needed for energy. It is stimulated by hormones such as glucagon and epinephrine, which are released when blood glucose levels are low.

In type 2 diabetes, glucose metabolism is impaired by insulin resistance and reduced insulin secretion. Insulin resistance prevents glucose from entering cells, especially in the muscles and fat tissues, which are the main sites of glucose uptake. This causes glucose to accumulate in the blood, leading to hyperglycemia (high blood sugar). Hyperglycemia, in turn, impairs the function of the pancreatic β-cells, which produce insulin. This results in reduced insulin secretion, which further worsens glucose metabolism. Moreover, insulin resistance and hyperglycemia affect the activity and expression of enzymes and genes involved in glucose metabolism, altering the balance between glycolysis, gluconeogenesis, and glycogenolysis. For example, insulin resistance and hyperglycemia increase gluconeogenesis and glycogenolysis, while decreasing glycolysis. This leads to increased glucose production and decreased glucose utilization, exacerbating the metabolic disorder.

The management of type 2 diabetes involves improving glucose metabolism by lowering blood glucose levels and increasing insulin sensitivity. This can be achieved by lifestyle modifications, such as diet, exercise, and weight loss, and by pharmacological interventions, such as oral antidiabetic drugs and insulin injections. Different drugs target different aspects of glucose metabolism, such as stimulating insulin secretion, enhancing insulin action, inhibiting glucose absorption, or reducing glucose production. The goal of treatment is to prevent or delay the onset of complications and improve the quality of life of people with type 2 diabetes.

CHAPTER 4

SIGNS AND SYMPTOMS

The following are a few typical type 2 diabetes symptoms and indicators::

- **Unusual thirst**: People with type 2 diabetes may feel more thirsty than usual because of the excess glucose in the blood, which draws water out of the cells and tissues. This can also cause dehydration and dry mouth.

- **Frequent urination**: The kidneys try to flush out the excess glucose from the blood by producing more urine. This can make a person need to urinate more often, especially at night.

- **Increased hunger**: People with type 2 diabetes may feel more hungry than usual because their cells are not getting enough glucose for energy. They may also experience cravings for sugary or starchy foods.

- **Fatigue**: People with type 2 diabetes may feel tired or weak because of the lack of glucose in the cells. They may also have difficulty concentrating or performing daily tasks.

- **Blurred vision**: High blood sugar levels can damage the small blood vessels in the eyes, which can affect the clarity of vision. This can also cause swelling of the lens, which can distort the vision. Permanent vision loss may result from this if treatment is not received.

- **Slow healing of cuts and wounds**: High blood sugar levels can impair the blood circulation and the immune system, which can affect the healing process of the skin. Cuts and wounds may take longer to heal and are more prone to infection.

- **Tingling, numbness, or pain in the hands or feet**: High blood sugar levels can damage the nerves, especially in the hands and feet. This can cause a loss of sensation or a feeling of pins and needles in the affected areas. This condition is called neuropathy and can worsen over time.

- **Dark patches of skin**: People with type 2 diabetes may develop areas of darkened skin, usually in the armpits, neck, or groin. This is caused by a condition called acanthosis nigricans, which is associated with insulin resistance.

These signs and symptoms may not be noticeable at first, or may be mild or intermittent. However, they can worsen over time and cause serious complications if not treated. Therefore, it is important to consult a doctor if you notice any of these signs and symptoms, or if you have risk factors for type 2 diabetes, such as obesity, family history, age, or prediabetes. A doctor can diagnose type 2 diabetes by performing blood tests to measure the blood sugar levels.

Type 2 diabetes can be managed by following a healthy diet, exercising regularly, taking medications, and monitoring the blood sugar levels. By doing so, people with type 2 diabetes can prevent or delay the onset of complications, such as heart disease, kidney failure, nerve damage, eye damage, or amputation.

• HYPERGLYCEMIA

Hyperglycemia is a condition where the blood sugar (glucose) level is higher than normal. It is a common and serious complication of type 2 diabetes, which occurs when the body does not use insulin properly or does not produce enough insulin. Hyperglycemia can damage various organs and tissues, such as the eyes, kidneys, nerves, and blood vessels, and increase the risk of heart disease and stroke.

Some of the causes of hyperglycemia in type 2 diabetes are:

- Eating too much or not following a balanced diet
- inadequate use of oral diabetes medicine or insulin
- Being physically inactive or not exercising regularly
- Having an infection, illness, injury, or surgery
- Experiencing stress, emotional problems, or hormonal changes

Some of the symptoms of hyperglycemia are[4]:

- Frequent urination and increased thirst

- Blurred vision and fatigue
- Headache and dry mouth
- Difficulty concentrating and irritability
- Fruity-smelling breath and nausea

If hyperglycemia is not treated promptly, it can lead to a life-threatening condition called ketoacidosis, which occurs when the body breaks down fat for energy and produces a high level of ketones, which are acidic substances that can make the blood too acidic. Ketoacidosis can cause symptoms such as:

- Abdominal pain and vomiting
- Shortness of breath and rapid breathing
- Confusion and loss of consciousness
- Coma and death

The treatment of hyperglycemia depends on the severity and the cause of the condition. Some of the general steps to lower blood sugar levels are:

- monitoring blood sugar levels frequently and documenting the findings
- Taking insulin or oral diabetes medications as prescribed by the doctor
- staying away from sugary drinks and consuming lots of water
- Eating healthy foods that are low in carbohydrates, fat, and salt

- Getting in at least 30 minutes of moderate exercise each day
- Seeing a doctor if symptoms worsen or don't go better

The prevention of hyperglycemia involves managing type 2 diabetes effectively and following a diabetes care plan that includes:

- Having regular check-ups with the doctor and getting blood tests to monitor blood sugar, cholesterol, and kidney function
- Following a personalized meal plan that meets the nutritional needs and preferences of the person
- Learning how to count carbohydrates and adjust insulin doses accordingly
- Using a glucose meter and a continuous glucose monitor to track blood sugar levels and trends
- Having a glucagon kit and a medical alert bracelet or necklace in case of emergencies
- Knowing the signs and symptoms of hyperglycemia and ketoacidosis and how to treat them
- Having a support system of family, friends, and health care professionals

who can help with diabetes management

Hyperglycemia is a serious complication of type 2 diabetes that can have long-term and life-threatening consequences. However, with proper care and education, people with type 2 diabetes can prevent and treat hyperglycemia and live healthy and fulfilling lives.

POLYURIA,POLYDIPSIA,AND POLYPHAGIA

One of the most common symptoms of type 2 diabetes is the three P's: polyuria, polydipsia, and polyphagia. These are medical terms that describe increased urination, thirst, and hunger, respectively. They are caused by the high blood glucose levels that result from insulin deficiency or resistance.

Polyuria means urinating more than normal, usually more than 3 liters per day. This happens because the kidneys try to remove the excess glucose from the blood by filtering more water along with it. This leads to frequent and large amounts of urine production, which can also cause dehydration and electrolyte imbalance.

Polydipsia means having an excessive and persistent thirst, even after drinking fluids. This is a response to the fluid loss and dehydration caused by polyuria. The brain senses the low water level in the body and signals the person to drink more. However, drinking more fluids can also worsen polyuria and create a vicious cycle.

Polyphagia means having an increased and abnormal appetite, especially for carbohydrates and sweets. This is due to the lack of glucose entering the cells, which makes them starved for energy. The body tries to compensate by increasing the hunger signal and craving more food. However, eating more food can also raise the blood glucose level and aggravate the condition.

The three P's of diabetes are not only unpleasant and inconvenient, but also dangerous if left untreated. They can lead to serious complications such as dehydration, ketoacidosis, weight loss, infections, kidney damage, and coma. Therefore, it is important to monitor the blood glucose level regularly and follow the treatment plan prescribed by the doctor. The treatment may include lifestyle changes, such as diet and exercise, and medications, such as oral drugs or insulin injections, to lower the blood glucose level and prevent or delay the complications of diabetes.

A. FATIGUE AND WEIGHT LOSS

Fatigue

Fatigue is a common symptom of type 2 diabetes. It can result from high or low blood sugar levels, dehydration, kidney damage, anemia, thyroid problems, or medication side effects Fatigue can also be caused by mental and emotional issues, such as depression or feeling overwhelmed by the diagnosis or complexity of medical care.

Fatigue can affect a person's quality of life and increase the risk of complications, such as infections, cardiovascular disease, or nerve damage. Therefore, it is important to identify and treat the underlying causes of fatigue, and to adopt healthy lifestyle habits that can boost energy levels. Some strategies to manage fatigue include:

- Monitoring and controlling blood sugar levels with medication, diet, and exercise
- Drinking enough water to prevent dehydration

- Getting regular check-ups to screen for and treat any diabetes-related complications or co-morbid conditions, such as kidney disease, anemia, or hypothyroidism
- Taking prescribed medications as directed and reporting any adverse effects to the doctor
- Getting enough sleep and following a consistent sleep schedule
- Reducing stress and seeking professional help for depression or anxiety if needed
- Engaging in physical activity that is appropriate for the level of fitness and health
- Eating a balanced diet that provides adequate nutrients and energy
- Seeking social support from family, friends, or support groups

Weight loss

Weight loss can also be a symptom of type 2 diabetes. It can occur when the body does not produce enough insulin or use it effectively, resulting in excess glucose in the blood. When this happens, the body starts burning fat and muscle for energy, causing a reduction in overall body weight[4] .

Weight loss can also be intentional, as part of a treatment plan to improve blood sugar control and reduce the risk of complications. Losing weight can help lower blood pressure, cholesterol, and triglyceride levels, and improve insulin sensitivity and cardiovascular health.

However, weight loss should be gradual and sustainable, and not compromise the nutritional needs of the body. Rapid or excessive weight loss can have negative effects, such as dehydration, electrolyte imbalance, gallstones, malnutrition, or muscle loss. Therefore, it is advisable to consult a doctor or a dietitian before starting a weight loss program, and to follow these general guidelines:

- Setting realistic and achievable goals, such as losing 5% to 10% of the initial body weight over 6 to 12 months
- Creating a calorie deficit of 500 to 1,000 calories per day, which can result in losing 1 to 2 pounds per week
- Choosing foods that are low in calories, fat, and sugar, and high in fiber, protein, and vitamins
- Eating smaller and more frequent meals, and avoiding skipping meals or fasting

- Drinking plenty of water and limiting the intake of alcohol and sugary drinks
- Increasing physical activity, aiming for at least 150 minutes of moderate-intensity exercise per week
- Monitoring weight and blood sugar levels regularly and adjusting the plan as needed
- Seeking support and motivation from health professionals, family, friends, or online communities

CHAPTER 5

DIAGNOSIS

DIAGNOSIS is the process of identifying the nature and cause of a certain illness or problem by examining the symptoms. It can also refer to the judgment or decision reached by this process. For example, a doctor may make a diagnosis of diabetes after testing a patient's blood sugar level. Diagnosis can help determine the appropriate treatment and prognosis for a patient.

BLOOD GLUCOSE TESTS

Blood glucose tests are used to diagnose and monitor type 2 diabetes, a condition that results from insufficient production of insulin or resistance to insulin, causing high blood sugar levels. There are different types of blood glucose tests, each with its own purpose and procedure. Here is a comprehensive overview of the main blood glucose tests:

- A1C test: This test calculates your blood sugar average over the previous two or three months. . It is also called the glycated hemoglobin test, because it reflects how much glucose is attached to the hemoglobin in your red blood cells. The A1C test does not require fasting or drinking any solution. It is done by taking a blood sample from a vein in your arm or a finger prick. The result is expressed as percentage.
- A1C readings under 5.7% are considered normal, those between 5.7 and 6.4% suggest prediabetes, while readings over 6.5% on two different tests indicate diabetes..

- **Fasting blood sugar test**: This test measures your blood sugar level after an overnight fast (not eating for at least 8 hours). It is also called the fasting plasma glucose test. It is done by taking a blood sample from a vein in your arm or a finger prick.Millimoles of sugar per liter (mmol/L) or milligrams of sugar per deciliter (mg/dL) are used to express the results. 99 mg/dL or less is considered normal during fasting; 100 to 125 mg/dL is indicative of prediabetes; and 126 mg/dL or more on two different tests is indicative of diabetes..

- **A glucose tolerance test:** analyzes your blood sugar levels both before and after consuming a glucose-containing beverage.. It is also called the oral glucose tolerance test or the OGTT. It is done by taking a blood sample from a vein in your arm or a finger prick before you drink the glucose solution.Your blood sugar will then be measured one, two, and maybe three hours after you consume the solution. The result is expressed in mg/dL or mmol/L of blood.Two hours later, 140 mg/dL or less is regarded as normal, 140 to 199 mg/dL as prediabetes, and 200 mg/dL or greater as diabetes.. The glucose tolerance test is usually used to diagnose gestational diabetes, a type of diabetes that develops during pregnancy.

- **Random blood sugar test**: This test measures your blood sugar level at the time you are tested. You can take this test at any time and do not need to fast or drink any solution. It is done by taking a blood sample from a vein in your arm or a finger prick. The result is expressed in mg/dL or mmol/L of blood. A blood sugar level of 200 mg/dL or higher, regardless of when you last ate, suggests diabetes, especially if you also have symptoms of diabetes, such as frequent urination and extreme thirst.

Blood glucose tests are important tools for diagnosing and managing type 2 diabetes. They can help you and your health care provider to determine your risk of developing diabetes, to confirm the diagnosis, to monitor your blood sugar level, to adjust your treatment plan, and to prevent or delay complications of diabetes. You should follow your health care provider's recommendations on how often and when to take these tests, as well as how to interpret the results and what actions to take based on them.

AIC TEST

The AIC test, also known as the A1C test, is a blood test that measures your average blood glucose levels over the past 3 months. It is used to diagnose and monitor type 2 diabetes and prediabetes. Here is some information about the AIC test and how it relates to type 2 diabetes:

- The AIC test is based on the amount of glucose that attaches to the hemoglobin proteins in your red blood cells.
- The component of a red blood cell that transports oxygen to the cells is called hemoglobin. The higher your blood glucose levels, the more glucose will bind to the hemoglobin. The AIC test result is reported as a percentage of hemoglobin with attached glucose.
- A normal AIC level is below 5.7%. A level of 5.7% to 6.4% indicates prediabetes, which means you have a higher risk of developing type 2 diabetes and cardiovascular disease. A level of 6.5% or more indicates diabetes.

- If you have risk factors for prediabetes or diabetes, such as being overweight, having a family history of diabetes, or being physically inactive, you should talk with your doctor about whether you should be tested. The AIC test does not require fasting, which means that blood can be drawn for the test at any time of the day.
- If you are diagnosed with type 2 diabetes, your doctor will use the AIC test to monitor your diabetes treatment plan and help you achieve your blood glucose goals. The AIC test can also help your doctor adjust your medication dosage or change your treatment if needed·
- The AIC test reflects your average blood glucose levels over the past 3 months, but it does not show the daily fluctuations or the effects of food, exercise, or medication on your blood glucose. Therefore, you should also use a blood glucose meter to check your blood glucose levels regularly and follow your doctor's advice on diet, physical activity, and medication.

- The AIC test can also be used to estimate your average blood glucose level, which is measured in milligrams per deciliter (mg/dL) or millimoles per liter (mmol/L). To convert your AIC percentage to an estimated average glucose level, you can use this formula: 28.7 x AIC - 46.7 = estimated average glucose.For example, if your AIC is 7%, your estimated average glucose is 154 mg/dL or 8.6 mmol/L.
- The AIC test is a useful tool for diagnosing and managing type 2 diabetes, but it is not perfect. Some factors can affect the accuracy of the AIC test, such as anemia, kidney disease, liver disease, pregnancy, or certain medications. Therefore, you should always discuss your AIC test results and your diabetes care plan with your doctor

DIAGNOSIS CRITERIA

Diagnosis criteria are the specific combination of signs, symptoms, and test results that a clinician uses to determine the correct diagnosis of a patient's condition[1] Diagnosis criteria can vary depending on the type and severity of the condition, as well as the diagnostic method used. For example, some common diagnosis criteria are:

- **DSM-5** for mental disorders: This is a manual that lists the criteria for different categories of mental disorders, such as autism spectrum disorder, schizophrenia, depression, etc. The criteria include observable behaviors, psychological symptoms, duration, and impact on functioning.
- **A1C** for diabetes: This is a blood test that measures the average level of glucose in the blood over the past three months. A higher A1C indicates a higher risk of diabetes and its complications. The diagnosis criteria for diabetes using A1C are:
    - An A1C of 6.5% or higher
    - An A1C of 5.7–6.4% indicates prediabetes
    - An A1C of less than 5.7% is normal
- **Amsterdam criteria** for hereditary nonpolyposis colorectal cancer: This is a set of criteria that helps identify families with a genetic predisposition to

colorectal cancer. The criteria include having at least three relatives with colorectal cancer, one of whom is a first-degree relative of the other two, and having at least one case of colorectal cancer diagnosed before age 50.

CHAPTER 6

COMPLICATIONS

Complications are unfavorable or harmful outcomes that result from a disease, condition, or treatment. They can make the situation more difficult, confusing, or dangerous. Complications can affect the prognosis or recovery of the patient. They can also lead to new or secondary diseases or problems.

Some examples of complications are:

- Infection after surgery
- Bleeding or clotting after an injury
- Kidney failure due to diabetes
- Stroke due to high blood pressure
- Pneumonia due to COVID-19

Complications can be prevented or reduced by following proper medical advice, taking precautions, and monitoring the condition. If complications occur, they should be treated promptly and appropriately.

CARDIOVASCULAR COMPLICATIONS

Cardiovascular complications are problems that affect the heart and blood vessels. They can result from various conditions, such as coronary artery disease, arrhythmias, congenital heart defects, and heart failure. Some of the common cardiovascular complications are:

- **Heart attack**: This occurs when a blood clot blocks the blood flow to the heart muscle, causing damage or death of the heart cells. Breathlessness, sweating, nausea, and chest pain are some of the symptoms.
- **Stroke**: This occurs when a blood clot blocks the blood flow to the brain, causing damage or death of the brain cells. Symptoms include numbness, weakness, confusion, trouble speaking, and loss of balance.
- **Pulmonary embolism**: This occurs when a blood clot travels to the lungs, blocking the blood flow and reducing the oxygen supply. Symptoms include shortness of breath, chest pain, coughing, and bluish skin.

- **Cardiac arrest**: This occurs when the heart stops beating suddenly, causing the blood flow to the body to stop. Symptoms include loss of consciousness, no pulse, and no breathing.
- **Peripheral artery disease**: This occurs when the blood vessels in the legs or arms are narrowed or blocked by plaque, reducing the blood flow and causing pain, numbness, or infection.
- **Atrial fibrillation**: This occurs when the upper chambers of the heart beat irregularly and fast, causing the blood to pool and form clots. Symptoms include palpitations, dizziness, fatigue, and chest discomfort.
- **Angina**: This occurs when the heart does not get enough oxygen due to narrowed or blocked coronary arteries. Symptoms include chest pain, pressure, or tightness that may radiate to the neck, jaw, or arm.

Cardiovascular complications can be life-threatening and require immediate medical attention. They can also lead to long-term effects, such as disability, reduced quality of life, and increased risk of other complications. Therefore, it is important to prevent and treat the underlying causes of cardiovascular complications, such as high blood pressure, high cholesterol, diabetes, smoking, obesity, and physical inactivity.

NEUROPATHY

Neuropathy refers to a condition where peripheral nerves, responsible for transmitting signals between the central nervous system and the rest of the body, are damaged. This can result in symptoms like pain, tingling, and numbness, often affecting the hands and feet. Causes include diabetes, autoimmune disorders, infections, and certain medications. Treatment aims to manage symptoms and address the underlying cause when possible.

RETINOPATHY

Retinopathy is a broad term referring to any non-inflammatory disorder of the retina, the light-sensitive layer at the back of the eye. It often occurs due to damage to blood vessels in the retina, impacting its function. There are various types of retinopathy, with diabetic retinopathy being one of the most common.

1. Diabetic Retinopathy:
    - Caused by prolonged high blood sugar levels damaging blood vessels in the retina.
    - Early stages may be asymptomatic, but as it progresses, it can lead to vision loss.
    - For early detection and treatment, routine eye exams are essential.
2. Hypertensive Retinopathy:
    - Associated with high blood pressure, causing damage to the small blood vessels in the retina.

- Symptoms may include blurred vision, headaches, or vision disturbances.
- Controlling blood pressure is key to preventing and managing hypertensive retinopathy.

3. Retinopathy of Prematurity (ROP):
- Affects premature infants, involving abnormal blood vessel development in the retina.
- Severity varies; severe cases can lead to retinal detachment and vision impairment.
- Monitoring and timely intervention are critical for managing ROP.

4. Radiation Retinopathy:
- Results from exposure to ionizing radiation, often during cancer treatment.
- Symptoms include vision changes, retinal hemorrhages, and swelling.
- Management involves addressing the underlying cause and symptomatic treatment.

5. Retinal Vein or Artery Occlusion:
- Occurs when blood vessels supplying the retina are blocked, leading to reduced blood flow.

- o Can cause sudden vision loss, depending on the affected vessels.
- o Treatment varies but may include addressing underlying vascular issues.
6. Symptoms and Diagnosis:
    - o Common symptoms include blurred vision, floaters, flashes of light, and vision loss.
    - o Diagnosis typically involves a comprehensive eye exam, including imaging studies like fundus photography and angiography.
7. Management and Treatment:
    - o The severity of the ailment and its underlying cause will determine how it is treated.
    - o Diabetic retinopathy may require laser therapy or injections to manage abnormal blood vessels.
    - o Hypertensive retinopathy often improves with blood pressure control.
    - o Regular eye exams and early intervention are crucial for preventing irreversible damage.

In summary, retinopathy encompasses various conditions affecting the retina, with causes ranging from diabetes and hypertension to prematurity and radiation exposure. Early detection and appropriate management are essential for preserving vision and preventing complications.

NEPHROPATHY

Nephropathy refers to damage or disease affecting the kidneys. It can manifest in various forms, with common types including diabetic nephropathy, hypertensive nephropathy, and glomerulonephritis.

1. Diabetic Nephropathy:

- Caused by prolonged diabetes, it damages the small blood vessels in the kidneys. Symptoms may include protein in urine, high blood pressure, and fluid retention.

2. Hypertensive Nephropathy:

- Over time, high blood pressure can harm the kidneys.It often leads to reduced blood flow, causing gradual impairment of kidney function.

3. Glomerulonephritis:

- Inflammation of the glomeruli, the kidney's filtering units. This can result from infections, autoimmune diseases, or other immune system abnormalities.

Common Symptoms:

- Persistent proteinuria (protein in urine)
- Hematuria (blood in urine)
- fluid retention causing swelling in the face, ankles, or legs
- Fatigue, weakness, and anemia

Diagnostic Methods:

- Urinalysis to detect abnormalities in urine
- Blood tests to determine blood urea nitrogen and creatinine levels
- imaging tests like CT or ultrasound scans
- Management and Treatment:
- Controlling underlying conditions like diabetes and hypertension
- medication to control the symptoms and halt the progression
- Dietary changes, including sodium and protein restriction
- Dialysis or kidney transplant in severe cases

Prevention:

- Regular monitoring for those at risk, such as diabetics and hypertensive individuals
- lifestyle adjustments, like eating a well-balanced diet and getting regular exercise
- Prompt treatment of infections to prevent glomerulonephritis

Complications:

- Chronic kidney disease (CKD)
- End-stage renal disease (ESRD)
- Cardiovascular complications due to fluid retention and electrolyte imbalances

Early detection and management are crucial in preventing further kidney damage. Individuals with risk factors should undergo regular check-ups and follow a healthy lifestyle to mitigate the chances of nephropathy development.

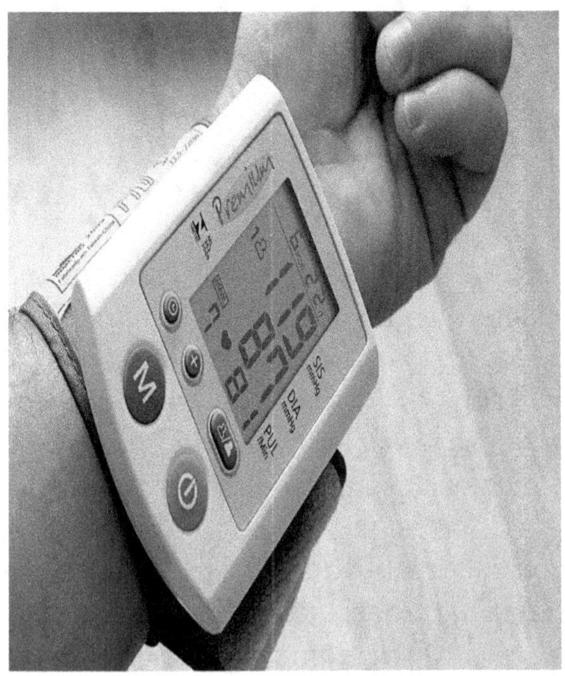

CHAPTER 7

MANAGEMENT AND TREATMENT

Type 2 diabetes is a chronic condition that affects how the body processes glucose, a type of sugar that is the main source of energy for cells. People with type 2 diabetes either do not produce enough insulin, a hormone that regulates glucose uptake, or are resistant to its effects. This leads to high blood sugar levels, which can cause various complications, such as heart disease, kidney damage, nerve damage, and vision loss.

Management and treatment of type 2 diabetes aim to keep blood sugar levels within a healthy range and prevent or delay complications. This calls for a mix of medicine, lifestyle modifications, and ongoing observation.. Here are some of the key aspects of managing and treating type 2 diabetes:

- Healthy eating. A balanced diet that is low in saturated fat, salt, and added sugar, and high in fiber, fruits, vegetables, and whole grains can help control blood sugar levels and lower the risk of cardiovascular problems. People with type 2 diabetes should also limit their intake of alcohol and carbohydrates, especially refined ones, as they can raise blood sugar levels quickly. A dietitian can help plan a personalized meal plan that suits one's preferences, goals, and medical conditions.

- Regular exercise. Physical activity can improve insulin sensitivity, lower blood pressure, reduce body fat, and enhance mood and well-being. People with type 2 diabetes should aim for at least 150 minutes of moderate to vigorous aerobic exercise per week, such as walking, cycling, or swimming, and two or more sessions of strength training per week, such as lifting weights or doing resistance exercises. They should also check their blood sugar levels before, during, and after exercise, and adjust their medication, food, and fluid intake accordingly.

- Weight loss. Being overweight or obese can increase insulin resistance and the risk of complications from type 2 diabetes. Losing weight can improve blood sugar control, lower blood pressure and cholesterol, and reduce the need for medication. A modest weight loss of 5% to 10% of body weight can have significant benefits for people with type 2 diabetes. Weight loss can be achieved by following a healthy diet and increasing physical activity, as well as by using medication or surgery in some cases.

- Medication. Depending on the severity of type 2 diabetes and the response to lifestyle changes, some people may need to take one or more medications to lower their blood sugar levels. There are several classes of drugs that work in different ways, such as stimulating the pancreas to produce more insulin, reducing the liver's glucose output, enhancing the cells' uptake of glucose, or increasing the excretion of glucose in urine. Some of the common medications for type 2 diabetes include metformin, sulfonylureas, meglitinides, DPP-4 inhibitors, GLP-1 receptor agonists, SGLT2 inhibitors, and insulin. The choice of medication depends on various factors, such as the individual's blood sugar levels, medical history, side effects, and preferences. The dosage and timing of medication may also need to be adjusted over time, based on blood sugar monitoring and other tests

- Blood sugar monitoring. Keeping track of blood sugar levels is essential for managing and treating type 2 diabetes. This can help assess the effectiveness of the treatment plan, identify any fluctuations or patterns, and make necessary changes to medication, diet, or exercise. People with type 2 diabetes can use a home blood glucose meter, a device that measures blood sugar from a drop of blood obtained by pricking the finger, to check their blood sugar levels at different times of the day. They can also use a continuous glucose monitor, a device that measures blood sugar from a sensor inserted under the skin, to get real-time readings and alerts. The frequency and timing of blood sugar testing depend on the individual's treatment goals, medication, and lifestyle. A common test that measures the average blood sugar level over the past two to three months is the A1C test, which is usually done at least twice a year by a health care provider.

- Complication screening. People with type 2 diabetes are at a higher risk of developing various complications, such as eye damage, kidney damage, nerve damage, foot problems, heart disease, stroke, and infections. To prevent or detect these complications early, people with type 2 diabetes should have regular check-ups and tests with their health care providers. These may include blood pressure, cholesterol, kidney function, urine albumin, eye exam, foot exam, dental exam, and flu and pneumonia vaccines. They should also report any symptoms or signs of complications, such as blurred vision, numbness, tingling, pain, swelling, or ulcers in the feet, chest pain, shortness of breath, or signs of infection.

Managing and treating type 2 diabetes can be challenging, but it can also improve one's quality of life and reduce the risk of serious complications. By following a healthy lifestyle, taking medication as prescribed, monitoring blood sugar levels, and screening for complications, people with type 2 diabetes can live well and stay healthy.

LIFESTYLE MODIFICATIONS

Lifestyle modifications are changes in habits and behaviors that can help people with type 2 diabetes manage their condition and prevent or delay complications. Some of the most important lifestyle modifications for type 2 diabetes are:

- **Eating a healthy diet**: A balanced diet that includes plenty of vegetables, fruits, whole grains, lean proteins, and healthy fats can help control blood sugar levels and prevent weight gain. Carbohydrates, which are found in foods like bread, rice, pasta, potatoes, and sweets, have the biggest impact on blood sugar levels. People with type 2 diabetes should limit their intake of refined carbohydrates, such as white bread, white rice, and sugary foods, and choose complex carbohydrates, such as whole grains, beans, and lentils, that are rich in fiber and nutrients. Fiber can help slow down the absorption of sugar and keep blood sugar levels more stable. People with type 2 diabetes should also avoid foods that are high in saturated fat, such as fatty meats, cheese, butter, and pastries, and opt for foods that contain unsaturated fat, such as fish, nuts, seeds, and olive oil. Saturated fat can increase the risk of heart disease, which is a common complication of diabetes. A simple way to plan a healthy meal is to use the plate method, which involves dividing a 9-inch plate into four sections: half of the plate for non-starchy vegetables, one quarter for lean protein, and one quarter for healthy carbohydrates.

- **Being physically active**: Physical activity can help lower blood sugar levels, improve insulin sensitivity, reduce blood pressure, lower cholesterol, and prevent or reduce excess weight. It can also improve mood, energy, and overall well-being. People with type 2 diabetes should aim for at least 150 minutes of moderate-intensity physical activity per week, or 75 minutes of vigorous-intensity physical activity per week, or a combination of both.Moderate-intensity physical activity means that the heart rate and breathing are slightly increased, but the person can still talk comfortably. Examples of moderate-intensity physical activity include brisk walking, cycling, swimming, dancing, and gardening. Vigorous-intensity physical activity means that the heart rate and breathing are significantly increased, and the person can only say a few words without pausing for breath. Examples of vigorous-intensity physical activity include jogging, running, skipping, aerobics, and playing sports. People with type 2 diabetes should also do some strength training exercises at least twice a week, such as lifting weights, using resistance bands, or doing bodyweight exercises, to build and maintain muscle mass and bone density. Before starting any physical activity program, people with type 2 diabetes should consult their healthcare provider and check their blood sugar levels before, during, and after exercise.

- **Losing weight if overweight or obese**: Excess weight can make it harder for the body to use insulin properly and increase the risk of developing type 2 diabetes or worsening its symptoms. Losing weight can help improve blood sugar control, lower blood pressure, reduce cholesterol, and lower the risk of heart disease and other complications. People with type 2 diabetes who are overweight or obese should aim to lose weight gradually, by about 5 to 10% of their initial weight over a period of one year. This can be achieved by following a healthy diet and being physically active, as described above. People with type 2 diabetes should avoid crash diets, fad diets, or extreme weight loss methods, as they can be harmful to their health and may cause fluctuations in blood sugar levels. People with type 2 diabetes should also monitor their weight regularly and seek professional advice if they have difficulty losing weight or maintaining a healthy weight.

- **Quitting smoking**: Smoking can increase the risk of developing type 2 diabetes and worsen its complications, such as heart disease, stroke, kidney disease, nerve damage, and eye problems. Smoking can also affect blood sugar levels and make it harder to control diabetes. Quitting smoking can lower the risk of these complications and improve blood sugar control, as well as provide other health benefits, such as improved lung function, blood circulation, and immune system. People with type 2 diabetes who smoke should seek help from their healthcare provider or a smoking cessation program to quit smoking as soon as possible.

- **Managing stress**: Stress can affect blood sugar levels and make it harder to manage diabetes. Stress can also trigger unhealthy behaviors, such as overeating, smoking, drinking alcohol, or skipping medications. People with type 2 diabetes should try to identify and cope with the sources of stress in their lives, such as work, family, finances, or health issues. Some effective ways to manage stress include relaxation techniques, such as deep breathing, meditation, yoga, or tai chi, physical activity, hobbies, social support, counseling, or therapy.
- **Taking medications as prescribed**: Medications can help people with type 2 diabetes control their blood sugar levels and prevent or delay complications. There are different types of medications for type 2 diabetes, such

as pills, injections, or insulin, that work in different ways to lower blood sugar levels. People with type 2 diabetes should follow their healthcare provider's instructions on how, when, and how much medication to take, and report any side effects or problems. People with type 2 diabetes should also check their blood sugar levels regularly, as advised by their healthcare provider, and keep a record of the results. This can help them and their healthcare provider adjust their medication doses and lifestyle changes as needed.

These lifestyle modifications can help people with type 2 diabetes improve their quality of life and reduce the risk of serious complications. However, they are not a substitute for regular medical care and follow-up. People with type 2 diabetes should see their healthcare provider regularly, at least every three to six months, to monitor their blood sugar levels, blood pressure, cholesterol, kidney function, eye health, and foot health. They should also get vaccinated against influenza and pneumococcal disease, and have regular dental check-ups and screenings for depression and other mental health issues. People with type 2 diabetes should also seek emergency care if they experience any signs or symptoms of diabetic ketoacidosis, such as nausea, vomiting, abdominal pain, fruity breath, confusion, or coma, or hyperosmolar hyperglycemic state, such as extreme thirst, dry mouth, frequent urination, high fever, weakness, or seizures .

DIET

A diet is the food and drink that a person or animal usually consumes, or a specific selection of food for health or weight-management reasons.
diet for type 2 diabetes is a healthy-eating plan that helps control blood sugar levels, manage weight, and prevent or treat complications. It involves eating nutritious foods in moderate amounts and at regular times, and limiting or avoiding foods that are high in sugar, fat, salt, or calories.

Some general principles of a diet for type 2 diabetes are:

- Consuming regular meals and snacks at regular intervals
- Choosing foods that are rich in fiber, protein, healthy fats, and low-glycemic carbohydrates
- Limiting foods that are high in sugar, saturated fat, trans fat, and sodium
- staying away from sugary drinks and consuming lots of water
- Reading nutrition labels and measuring portion sizes

Some examples of foods to eat for type 2 diabetes are:

- Vegetables, such as broccoli, carrots, greens, peppers, tomatoes, potatoes, and corn
- Fruits, such as apples, avocado, berries, cherries, grapefruit, peaches, pears, and plums
- Whole grains include brown rice, quinoa, barley, oats, and whole wheat.
- Beans and legumes, such as black beans, lentils, kidney beans, chickpeas, and soybeans
- dairy products. such cottage cheese, yogurt, cheese, and low-fat milk
- Fish and seafood, such as tuna, salmon, sardines, mackerel, cod, and shrimp
- Lean meats including pig, turkey, chicken, and lean beef
- Nuts and seeds, including flax, sunflower, walnut, pecan, and almond
- Healthy fats, such as olive oil, canola oil, peanut oil, avocado, and nuts
- Herbs and spices, such as garlic, ginger, turmeric, cinnamon, and basil

Some examples of foods to limit or avoid for type 2 diabetes are:

- Sugar-filled beverages, like juice, soda, sports drinks, and energy drinks
- Sweets and desserts, such as candy, chocolate, ice cream, cakes, pies, and cookies
- Refined carbohydrates, such as white bread, white rice, white pasta, and pastries
- Processed foods, such as chips, crackers, pretzels, and popcorn

- Fried foods include doughnuts, onion rings, chicken nuggets, and french fries.
- High-fat dairy products, such as whole milk, cream, butter, and cheese
- Fatty meats, such as bacon, sausage, hot dogs, and ribs
- Trans fats, such as margarine, shortening, and baked goods
- Salt and sodium, such as salt, soy sauce, pickles, and canned foods
- Fast food, such as burgers, pizza, tacos, and sandwiches
- foods

A diet for type 2 diabetes should also include drinking plenty of water, avoiding alcohol or drinking in moderation, and choosing sugar-free or low-calorie options when possible.

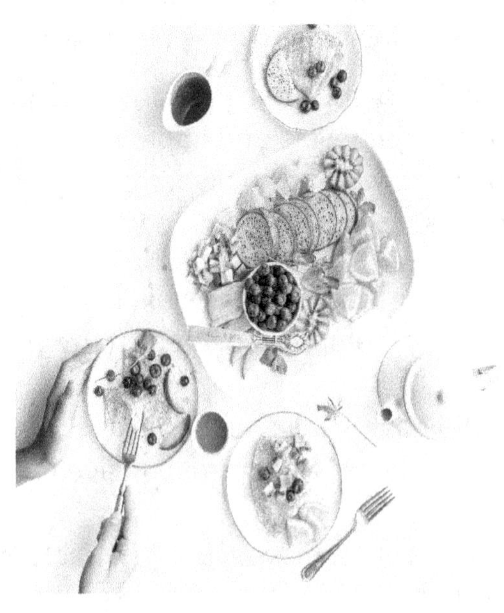

EXERCISE

Exercise is an important part of managing type 2 diabetes, as it can help lower blood sugar levels, reduce excess body weight, and improve overall health and well-being

Exercise is one of the best ways to manage your blood sugar levels and improve your overall health and well-being if you have type 2 diabetes. Exercise can help you:

- Lower your blood sugar levels by increasing the uptake of glucose by your muscles
- Improve your insulin sensitivity by making your cells more responsive to insulin
- Reduce your cardiovascular risk factors by lowering your blood pressure, cholesterol, and triglycerides
- Promote weight loss or maintenance by burning calories and increasing your metabolism
- Strengthen your muscles, bones, and joints by improving your muscle mass, bone density, and joint health
- Enhance your mood and self-esteem by releasing endorphins and reducing stress

- Improve your quality of life by increasing your energy, flexibility, and mobility

The American Diabetes Association (ADA) recommends that people with type 2 diabetes get at least 150 minutes of moderate-intensity aerobic exercise per week, spread over at least three days, with no more than two consecutive days without exercise. Aerobic exercise is any activity that makes your heart beat faster and your lungs work harder, such as walking, cycling, swimming, or dancing. The ADA also suggests doing resistance training at least twice a week, targeting all major muscle groups. Resistance training is any activity that makes your muscles work against a force, such as lifting weights, using resistance bands, or doing body-weight

exercises. Additionally, the ADA advises doing flexibility exercises, such as stretching, yoga, or pilates, to improve your range of motion and prevent injuries.

However, not all exercises are equally suitable for people with type 2 diabetes. Some exercises may be more appropriate for different fitness levels, preferences, and goals. In this article, we will explore the different types of exercise that can help you manage your type 2 diabetes, and provide some tips and precautions and on how to choose the best exercise for you.

Types of Exercise for Type 2 Diabetes

There are three main types of exercise that can benefit people with type 2 diabetes: aerobic, resistance, and flexibility exercises.
Here is a comprehensive definition of each exercise modality:

- **Aerobic exercise** is any activity that increases your heart rate and breathing for a sustained period of time, such as walking, biking, swimming, or dancing. Aerobic exercise helps to improve insulin sensitivity, lower blood glucose levels, reduce cardiovascular risk factors, and enhance mood and well-being.

- **Resistance exercise** is any activity that involves contracting your muscles against an external force, such as lifting weights, doing body-weight exercises, or using resistance bands. Resistance exercise helps to increase muscle mass, strength, and endurance, which can

improve glucose uptake, lower blood pressure, and prevent muscle loss·
- **Flexibility exercise** is any activity that stretches your muscles and joints, such as yoga, pilates, or tai chi. Flexibility exercise helps to improve range of motion, posture, balance, and coordination, which can prevent injuries, reduce pain, and enhance physical function·

Some examples of aerobic, resistance, and flexibility exercises that can be done at home are:

- **Aerobic exercise**: walking, jogging, skipping, jumping jacks, stair climbing, cycling, or using an elliptical machine.
- **Resistance exercise**: squats, lunges, push-ups, planks, dips, curls, rows, or using dumbbells, kettlebells, or resistance bands.
- **Flexibility exercise**: neck stretch, shoulder stretch, chest stretch, back stretch, hamstring stretch, calf stretch, or following a yoga, pilates, or tai chi video.

TIPS AND PRECAUTION

Exercises tips and benefits:-

- **Walking**: Walking is a simple and low-impact exercise that can be done anywhere and anytime. It can help increase insulin sensitivity, lower blood pressure, and improve cardiovascular health. Aim for at least 150 minutes of moderate-intensity walking per week, or 30 minutes five days a week. You can start slowly and gradually increase your pace and distance. Wear comfortable shoes and socks, and check your feet for blisters or injuries after each walk.
- **Cycling**: Cycling is another low-impact exercise that can help people with type 2 diabetes and joint pain. It can also improve blood glucose control, lower triglyceride levels, and reduce cardiovascular risk. With a stationary bike, you may ride both indoors and outside.Start with 10 to 15 minutes of cycling at a moderate intensity, and gradually increase the duration and intensity as you get fitter. Make sure your bike is well-adjusted and wear a helmet and reflective clothing if you cycle outside.
- **Swimming**: Swimming is a great exercise for people with type 2 diabetes, as it works the whole body without

putting stress on the joints. It can also lower blood sugar levels, blood pressure, and cholesterol levels. You can swim in a pool, a lake, or the ocean, as long as the water is clean and safe. Start with 10 minutes of swimming at a comfortable pace, and gradually increase the time and speed as you improve. Warm up before swimming and cool down after. Avoid swimming alone or in cold water, and wear goggles and ear plugs if needed.

- **Team sports**: Team sports can be fun and motivating, as they provide social interaction and a sense of commitment. They can also improve blood glucose control, aerobic fitness, and mental health. Some examples of team sports are basketball, soccer, softball, and tennis. Choose a sport that you enjoy and that suits your skill level. Join a recreational league or a group of friends who play regularly. Follow the rules and safety guidelines of the sport, and wear appropriate equipment and clothing. Monitor your blood sugar before, during, and after the game, and adjust your medication and food intake accordingly.

- **Aerobic dance**: Aerobic dance is a type of exercise that combines dance and aerobic movements for a fast-paced and fun workout. It can help lower blood sugar levels, blood pressure, and A1C levels. It can also improve mood, balance, and coordination. You can join an aerobic dance class, such as Zumba, or follow a video at home. Start with a low-impact and beginner-level class, and gradually progress to a higher-impact and advanced-level class. Sip lots of water, dress comfortably, and wear shoes that fit well.Stop if you feel dizzy, breathless, or chest pain.
- **Weightlifting**: Weightlifting is a type of resistance exercise that involves lifting weights or using machines to strengthen the muscles. It can help increase muscle mass and strength, which can improve blood glucose control and metabolism. It can also prevent muscle loss and osteoporosis, which are common in older adults with diabetes. You can lift weights at a gym, at home, or outdoors. Start with light weights and low repetitions, and gradually increase the weight and number of repetitions as you get stronger. Learn the proper

technique and form from a trainer or a video, and rest for at least one day between sessions. Avoid holding your breath or straining too hard, and check your blood pressure before and after lifting.

- **Resistance band exercises**: Resistance band exercises are another type of resistance exercise that use elastic bands to create tension and resistance for the muscles. They can help improve blood glucose control, muscle strength, and flexibility. They can also be done anywhere and anytime, as they are portable and easy to use. You can buy resistance bands online or at a sports store, and follow a video or a guide for different exercises. Start with a light or medium resistance band, and gradually move to a heavier one as you get stronger. Perform 8 to 12 repetitions of each exercise, and rest for one minute between sets. Do two to three sets of each exercise, two to three times a week. Stretch before and after each session, and stop if you feel pain or discomfort.
- **Calisthenics**: Calisthenics are exercises that use your own body

weight as resistance, such as push-ups, squats, lunges, and planks. They can help improve blood glucose control, muscle strength, and endurance. They can also be done anywhere and anytime, as they do not require any equipment. You can follow a video or a guide for different calisthenics exercises, and modify them according to your fitness level. Start with 10 to 15 minutes of calisthenics, and gradually increase the duration and intensity as you get fitter. Do calisthenics two to three times a week, and rest for at least one day between sessions. Breathe normally and keep your core tight during each exercise, and stop if you feel pain or discomfort.

- **Pilates**: Pilates is a type of exercise that focuses on core strength, posture, balance, and flexibility. It can help lower blood sugar levels, blood pressure, and stress.Additionally, it can enhance digestion, respiration, and mental clarity. You can do pilates on a mat or on a machine called a reformer, either at a studio or at home. Start with a beginner-level class or video, and gradually progress to a higher-level one as you improve. Wear comfortable clothes and socks, and use a cushion or a towel if needed. Do pilates two to three times a week, and rest for at least one day between sessions. Breathe deeply and smoothly during each exercise, and stop if you feel pain or discomfort.

- **Yoga**: Yoga is a type of exercise that combines physical poses, breathing techniques, and meditation. It can help lower blood sugar levels, blood pressure, and stress. It can also improve flexibility, balance, and mental health. You can do yoga at a studio or at home, either on a mat or on a chair. Start with a gentle or beginner-level class or video, and gradually progress to a more challenging one as you get more flexible and confident. Wear comfortable clothes and shoes, and use a block or a strap if needed. Do yoga two to three times a week, and rest for at least one day between sessions. Breathe deeply and calmly during each pose, and stop if you feel pain or discomfort.

Some general tips and precautions for exercising with type 2 diabetes are:

- Check with your doctor before starting any new exercise program, especially if you have any other health conditions or complications.
- Monitor your blood sugar levels before, during, and after exercise, and adjust your medication, food, and fluid intake accordingly. Carry a fast-acting carbohydrate source, such as glucose tablets or juice, in case of hypoglycemia (low blood sugar).
- Drink plenty of water before, during, and after exercise, and avoid alcohol and caffeine, as they can cause dehydration and affect blood sugar levels.
- Wear comfortable and appropriate clothing, shoes, and accessories for the type and weather of exercise. Protect yourself from the sun, heat, cold, and wind, and avoid exercising in extreme temperatures or humidity.
- Warm up for at least 10 minutes before exercise, and cool down for at least 10 minutes after exercise, to prevent injuries and complications.
- Listen to your body and exercise at your own pace and level. Do not overdo it or push yourself too hard, as this can cause stress and harm to your body.

Stop if you feel any symptoms of distress, such as chest pain, shortness of breath, dizziness, nausea, or headache, and seek medical attention if needed.

- Enjoy your exercise and have fun. Choose activities that you like and that suit your lifestyle and preferences. Invite a friend or a family member to join you for support and motivation. Set realistic and specific goals, and reward yourself for your achievements.

How to Select Your Ideal Workout

The best exercise for you depends on several factors, such as your current fitness level, health status, availability, and motivation. Here are some tips on how to choose the best exercise for you:

- Assess your fitness level. Before starting any exercise program, it is important to know your current fitness level, and set realistic and specific goals. You can use a simple test, such as the 6-minute walk test or the 1.5-mile run test, to measure your aerobic

fitness. You can also use a scale, a tape measure, or a body fat analyzer to assess your body composition. Additionally, you may speak with your physician or a trained
- fitness trainer to help you evaluate your fitness level and design a personalized exercise plan for you.
- Consider your health status. If you have type 2 diabetes, you may also have other health conditions or complications that may affect your ability to exercise. For example, if you have heart disease, you may need to limit the intensity and duration of your exercise, and monitor your heart rate and blood pressure. If you have nerve damage, you may need to avoid exercises that put pressure on your feet, and check your feet regularly for blisters, cuts, or infections. If you have eye problems, you may need to avoid exercises that increase the pressure in your eyes, such as lifting heavy weights or bending over. If you have any health concerns, you should talk to your doctor before starting or changing your exercise
- routine, and follow their advice and recommendations.

- Choose an exercise that you enjoy. One of the most important factors for sticking to an exercise program is enjoyment. If you enjoy the exercise that you do, you are more likely to do it regularly and consistently. You can choose an exercise that suits your personality, preferences, and interests. For example, if you like socializing, you can join a team sport, a fitness class, or a walking group. If you like being outdoors, you can go for a hike, a bike ride, or a swim. If you like variety, you can try different exercises, or mix and match them. The key is to find an exercise that makes you happy and motivated.
- Be flexible and adaptable. Sometimes, you may encounter obstacles or challenges that prevent you from doing your planned exercise. For example, you may have a busy schedule, bad weather, or an injury. Instead of giving up or skipping your exercise, you can be flexible and adaptable, and find alternative ways to stay active. For example, you can do a home workout, use an indoor bike or treadmill, or do some stretching or yoga. You can also adjust the intensity, duration, or

frequency of your exercise, depending on your situation and how you feel. The important thing is to keep moving and not let anything stop you from exercising.

Exercise is one of the best ways to manage type 2 diabetes and improve your quality of life. By following the above types, tips, and precautions, you can make exercise a safe and enjoyable part of your daily routine.

MEDICATIONS

Type 2 diabetes is a chronic condition that affects how the body metabolizes glucose, the main source of energy for the body. People with type 2 diabetes either have insulin resistance or do not produce enough insulin to maintain normal blood sugar levels.

There are many medications available to help manage type 2 diabetes. These medications work in different ways to lower blood sugar levels. Some of the common classes of medications for type 2 diabetes are:

- **Metformin**. This is usually the first medication prescribed for type 2 diabetes. It belongs to a class of drugs called biguanides, which lower blood sugar by reducing the amount of glucose produced by the liver and improving the sensitivity of the body tissues to insulin.
- **Sulfonylureas**. These are oral medications that belong to a class of drugs called secretagogues, which stimulate the pancreas to produce and release more insulin. Examples of

sulfonylureas are glipizide, glimepiride, and glyburide

- **Meglitinides**. These are also oral medications that belong to the class of secretagogues, but they act faster and for a shorter duration than sulfonylureas. They are taken before meals to trigger a burst of insulin. Repaglinide and Nateglinide are two examples of meglitinides.
- **Thiazolidinediones**. These are oral medications that belong to a class of drugs called peroxisome proliferator-activated receptor gamma (PPAR-gamma) agonists, which increase the sensitivity of the body tissues to insulin and lessen the quantity of glucose the liver releases. Pioglitazone and rosiglitazone are two examples of thiazolidinediones.
- **Dipeptidyl peptidase-4 (DPP-4) inhibitors**. These are oral medications that belong to a class of drugs called incretin enhancers, which increase the level of a hormone called glucagon-like peptide-1 (GLP-1) that helps lower blood sugar by promoting the production of insulin and preventing the secretion of glucagon. . Examples of DPP-4

inhibitors are sitagliptin, saxagliptin, linagliptin, and alogliptin.

- **Sodium-glucose cotransporter 2 (SGLT2) inhibitors**. These are oral medications that belong to a class of drugs called gliflozins, which lower blood sugar by preventing the kidneys from reabsorbing glucose and increasing the amount of glucose excreted in urine. Canagliflozin, dapagliflozin, and empagliflozin are a few examples of SGLT2 inhibitors.
- **GLP-1 receptor agonists**. These are injectable medications that belong to a class of drugs called incretin mimetics, which mimic the action of GLP-1 and lower blood sugar by stimulating insulin secretion, inhibiting glucagon secretion, slowing gastric emptying, and reducing appetite. Examples of GLP-1 receptor agonists are liraglutide, semaglutide, tirzepatide, exenatide, and dulaglutide.
- **Insulin**. This is a hormone that is essential for regulating blood sugar levels. People with type 2 diabetes may need to take insulin injections if their blood sugar levels are not controlled by other medications or lifestyle changes. There are different types of insulin, such

as rapid-acting, short-acting, intermediate-acting, and long-acting, that vary in how quickly and how long they work.

The choice of medication for type 2 diabetes depends on several factors, such as the severity of the condition, the patient's preferences, the cost and availability of the drugs, and the potential side effects and interactions. Some people may need to take more than one medication to achieve optimal blood sugar control. It is important to consult with a doctor before starting, changing, or stopping any medication for type 2 diabetes.

INSULIN THERAPY

Insulin therapy is a treatment option for people with type 2 diabetes who have difficulty controlling their blood sugar levels with oral medications and lifestyle changes. Insulin is a hormone that helps the body use glucose (sugar) from food for energy or store it for future use. People with type 2 diabetes either do not produce enough insulin or their cells are resistant to its action, resulting in high blood sugar levels. Insulin therapy can help lower blood sugar levels and prevent or delay diabetes complications, such as heart disease, kidney disease, eye problems, and nerve damage.

There are different types of insulin that vary in how quickly they start working, how long they last, and when they peak. They can be classified into four categories: rapid-acting, short-acting, intermediate-acting, and long-acting. Rapid-acting and short-acting insulins are used to cover meals and correct high blood sugar levels. Intermediate-acting and long-acting insulins are used to provide basal (background) insulin throughout the day and night. Some insulins are premixed, meaning they contain a combination of two types of insulin in one vial or pen.

Insulin therapy can be initiated as augmentation or replacement. Augmentation means adding insulin to oral medications, while replacement means switching to insulin only. The choice of insulin regimen depends on several factors, such as the patient's blood sugar levels, preferences, lifestyle, and ability to self-monitor and self-inject. Some common insulin regimens are:

- Basal insulin plus oral medications. This regimen involves taking one injection of long-acting or intermediate-acting insulin once or twice a day, along with oral medications. This can be a simple and effective way to start insulin therapy for patients with type 2 diabetes who have high fasting blood sugar levels but relatively normal post-meal levels.
- Basal-bolus insulin. This regimen involves taking multiple injections of rapid-acting or short-acting insulin before each meal, plus one injection of long-acting or intermediate-acting insulin once or twice a day. This mimics the natural pattern of insulin secretion and allows for more flexibility and accuracy

in dosing. This is considered the most intensive and effective insulin regimen, but it also requires more monitoring and education.

- Premixed insulin. This regimen involves taking one or two injections of premixed insulin per day, usually before breakfast and dinner. Premixed insulin contains a fixed ratio of rapid-acting or short-acting insulin and intermediate-acting insulin. This can be a convenient and simple way to start insulin therapy for patients with type 2 diabetes who have high blood sugar levels throughout the day, but it also limits the ability to adjust the doses of each insulin component separately.
- Insulin pump. This is a device that delivers continuous subcutaneous infusion of rapid-acting or short-acting insulin through a thin tube and a small needle inserted under the skin. The pump can be programmed to deliver different amounts of insulin at different times of the day, depending on the patient's needs. The pump also allows the patient to deliver extra doses of insulin (boluses) before meals or to correct high blood sugar levels. This can

provide more flexibility and control over blood sugar levels, but it also requires more training and maintenance.

The dose of insulin is determined by the patient's weight, blood sugar levels, carbohydrate intake, physical activity, and other factors. The dose may need to be adjusted over time, depending on the patient's response and goals. The dose can be calculated using various methods, such as:

- Rule of thumb. This is a simple method that involves multiplying the patient's weight in kilograms by 0.3 to 1.0 to get the total daily dose of insulin in units. The total daily dose can then be divided into basal and bolus doses, depending on the insulin regimen. For example, a patient who weighs 70 kg and needs 0.6 unit per kg per day would need a total of 42 units of insulin per day. If the patient is on a basal-bolus regimen, he or she could take 50% of the total dose as basal insulin and 50% as bolus insulin, meaning 21 units of basal insulin and 7 units of bolus insulin before each meal.
- Sliding scale. This is a method that involves adjusting the dose of rapid-acting or short-acting insulin

before each meal or snack, based on the patient's blood sugar level at that time. The patient follows a table or chart that specifies how much insulin to take for different ranges of blood sugar levels. For example, a patient who has a blood sugar level of 180 mg/dL before breakfast could take 4 units of rapid-acting insulin, according to the following sliding scale:

Table

Blood sugar level (mg/dL)	Insulin dose (units)
Less than 70	0
70 to 120	2
121 to 180	4
181 to 240	6

241 to 300   8

More than 300   10

- Carbohydrate counting. This is a method that involves estimating the amount of carbohydrates in each meal or snack, and taking a dose of rapid-acting or short-acting insulin that matches the carbohydrate intake. The patient needs to know the carbohydrate content of different foods and beverages, and use a formula to calculate the insulin dose. The formula involves two factors: the insulin-to-carbohydrate ratio and the correction factor. The insulin-to-carbohydrate ratio is the number of grams of carbohydrates covered by one unit of insulin. The correction factor is the amount that one unit of insulin lowers the blood sugar level. For example, a patient who has an insulin-to-carbohydrate ratio of 1:15 and a correction factor of 50 could take the following dose of rapid-acting insulin before breakfast:

Table

Item	Carbohydrate content (g)
2 slices of toast	30
1 cup of milk	12
1 banana	27
Total	69

Insulin dose = (Carbohydrate intake / Insulin-to-carbohydrate ratio) + (Blood sugar level - Target blood sugar level / Correction factor)

If the patient's blood sugar level before breakfast is 200 mg/dL and the target blood sugar level is 120 mg/dL, the insulin dose would be:

Insulin dose = (69 / 15) + (200 - 120 / 50) = 4.6 + 1.6 = 6.2 units

The patient could round up the dose to 7 units of rapid-acting insulin.

Insulin therapy requires careful monitoring and education to ensure safety and effectiveness. The patient needs to check his or her blood sugar levels regularly, using a glucose meter or a continuous glucose monitor, and record the results. The patient also needs to learn how to recognize and treat low blood sugar levels (hypoglycemia), which can occur if the insulin dose is too high, the carbohydrate intakeis either too low or too excessive in terms of physical activity. Symptoms of hypoglycemia include sweating, shaking, hunger, dizziness, confusion, and weakness. Hypoglycemia can be treated by consuming 15 to 20 grams of fast-acting carbohydrates, such as glucose tablets, juice, or candy, and rechecking the blood sugar level after 15 minutes. If the blood sugar level is still low, the patient should repeat the treatment until the blood sugar level is normal.

The patient also needs to learn how to prevent and treat high blood sugar levels (hyperglycemia), which can occur if the insulin dose is too low, the carbohydrate intake is too high, or the physical activity is too low. Symptoms of hyperglycemia include thirst, frequent urination, blurred vision, fatigue, and nausea. Hyperglycemia can be treated by taking extra doses of insulin, as prescribed by the health care provider, and drinking plenty of fluids. If the blood sugar level is very high or the patient has signs of diabetic ketoacidosis, such as fruity breath, abdominal pain, vomiting, or difficulty breathing, the patient should seek emergency medical attention.

Insulin therapy can improve the quality of life and health outcomes of people with type 2 diabetes, but it also requires commitment and support from the patient and the health care team. The patient should work closely with the health care provider to choose the best insulin regimen, dose, and delivery method, and to adjust them as needed. The patient should also follow a healthy diet, exercise regularly, and attend regular check-ups and education sessions. By doing so, the patient can achieve optimal blood sugar control and reduce the risk of diabetes complications.

CHAPTER 8

PREVENTION

The good news is that you can prevent or delay the onset of type 2 diabetes and lower your risk of heart disease by making some lifestyle changes. Here are some tips to help you:

- **Maintain a healthy weight.** Being overweight or obese can make your body resistant to insulin, a hormone that regulates blood sugar levels. Losing weight can improve your insulin sensitivity and lower your blood pressure and cholesterol levels, which are all risk factors for heart disease. Aim for a body mass index (BMI) between 18.5 and 24.9, and a waist circumference of less than 40 inches for men and less than 35 inches for women.
- **Eat a balanced diet.** Choose foods that are low in saturated fat, trans fat, cholesterol, salt, and added sugars. Eat more fruits, vegetables, whole grains, lean protein, and healthy fats. Limit your intake of red meat, processed meat, refined carbohydrates, and sugary

drinks. A good example of a healthy eating plan is the DASH diet, which is designed to lower blood pressure and prevent heart disease.

- **Be physically active.** Exercise can help you control your blood sugar, blood pressure, and cholesterol levels, as well as reduce stress and improve your mood. Aim for at least 150 minutes of moderate-intensity aerobic activity (such as brisk walking, cycling, or swimming) or 75 minutes of vigorous-intensity aerobic activity (such as running, jumping rope, or playing sports) per week. You can also do some strength training (such as lifting weights, doing push-ups, or using resistance bands) at least twice a week to build muscle and bone health.
- **Quit smoking.** Smoking can damage your blood vessels and increase your risk of heart disease and stroke. It can also make it harder to control your blood sugar and worsen your diabetes complications. If you smoke, talk to your doctor about ways to quit. There are many options available, such as nicotine patches, gum, lozenges, inhalers, sprays, medications, and counseling.

- **Limit alcohol.** Drinking too much alcohol can raise your blood pressure, triglycerides, and blood sugar levels, as well as damage your liver and pancreas. It can also interfere with your diabetes medications and increase your risk of hypoglycemia (low blood sugar). If you choose to drink, do so in moderation. That means no more than one drink per day for women and two drinks per day for men. One drink is equivalent to 12 ounces of beer, 5 ounces of wine, or 1.5 ounces of liquor.
- **Manage stress.** Stress can affect your blood sugar, blood pressure, and heart health. It can also make you more likely to overeat, smoke, drink, or skip exercise. To cope with stress, try to find healthy ways to relax and unwind, such as meditation, yoga, breathing exercises, hobbies, or spending time with friends and family. You can also seek professional help from a therapist, counselor, or support group if you feel overwhelmed or depressed.
- **Monitor your blood sugar.** Keeping your blood sugar within a healthy range can prevent or delay the damage that diabetes can cause to your heart and

other organs. You can check your blood sugar at home using a glucose meter, or wear a continuous glucose monitor (CGM) that tracks your blood sugar levels throughout the day. Your doctor will tell you how often and when to test your blood sugar, and what your target range should be. You can also get an A1C test every 3 to 6 months to measure your average blood sugar level over the past 2 to 3 months.

- **Take your medications.** Depending on your condition, your doctor may prescribe you medications to help you control your blood sugar, blood pressure, and cholesterol levels. These medications can reduce your risk of heart disease and other diabetes complications, but only if you take them as directed. Follow your doctor's instructions on how, when, and how much to take your medications, and do not stop or change them without consulting your doctor. Tell your doctor about any side effects or problems you have with your medications, and ask about any interactions with other drugs, supplements, or foods.

- **See your doctor regularly.** Having regular check-ups with your doctor can help you monitor your diabetes and heart health, and prevent or treat any problems that may arise. Your doctor can also adjust your treatment plan as needed, and provide you with education and support. You should see your doctor at least once a year, or more often if you have any concerns or complications. You should also see other health care professionals, such as a diabetes educator, a dietitian, an eye doctor, a dentist, a podiatrist, and a cardiologist, as recommended by your doctor.

By following these tips, you can prevent or manage type 2 diabetes and lower your risk of heart disease. Remember, you are not alone in this journey. You can find support and resources from your health care team, your family and friends, and various organizations and communities. Together, you can live a healthy and happy life with diabetes.

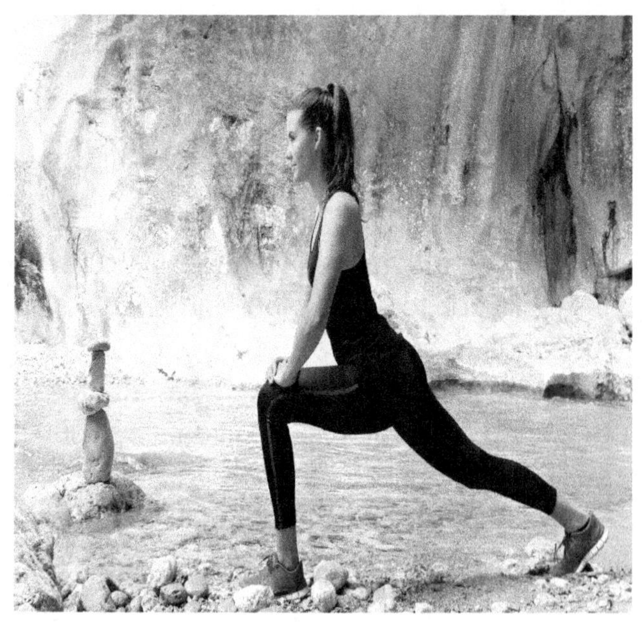

CHAPTER 9

LIVING WITH TYPE 2 DIABETES

Living with type 2 diabetes involves maintaining a balanced lifestyle. It includes regular monitoring of blood sugar levels, adopting a healthy diet rich in whole foods, managing weight through exercise, and taking prescribed medications. Additionally, regular check-ups with healthcare professionals are crucial for managing and adjusting the treatment plan. Emotional well-being plays a role too, as coping with the diagnosis and stress management are important aspects of overall health.

COPING STRATEGIES

Coping with type 2 diabetes involves adopting a multifaceted approach that includes lifestyle changes, medication adherence, and emotional well-being. Here are comprehensive coping strategies:

1. Stress Management: Prolonged stress might have an effect on blood sugar levels. . Practice stress-reducing techniques such as meditation, deep breathing, yoga, or mindfulness to maintain emotional well-being.
2. Weight Management: Achieving and maintaining a healthy weight can significantly impact diabetes management. Even modest weight loss can improve insulin sensitivity and overall health.
3. Educate Yourself: Understand the basics of diabetes, its complications, and how lifestyle choices impact the condition. Attend educational sessions, read reliable sources, and stay informed about advancements in diabetes management.
4. Regular Medical Check-ups: Schedule regular check-ups with healthcare professionals to monitor overall health and address any emerging issues promptly. Regular eye exams, foot checks, and screenings for complications are essential.
5. Support System: Build a strong support network with family, friends, and healthcare providers. Share your concerns, seek guidance, and involve loved ones in your diabetes management journey.
6. Goal Setting: Set realistic and achievable goals related to diet, exercise, and overall health. Breaking down larger objectives into

smaller, manageable steps can make the process more sustainable.
7. Stay Hydrated: Adequate hydration is essential for people with diabetes. Water helps regulate blood sugar levels and supports overall health.
8. Sleep Hygiene: Prioritize sufficient and quality sleep. Lack of sleep can negatively impact blood sugar control and contribute to overall health issues.

Remember, individualized approaches may vary, so it's crucial to work closely with healthcare professionals to tailor coping strategies to your specific needs and circumstances.

SUPPORT SYSTEM

A comprehensive support system for individuals with Type 2 diabetes involves various components to address their physical, emotional, and educational needs.

1. Medical Care:

- ○ Regular check-ups with healthcare professionals, including endocrinologists, dietitians, and primary care physicians, are essential.
- ○ Medication management and adjustments as needed should be monitored closely.

2. Nutritional Guidance:
   - ○ Collaboration with a registered dietitian for personalized meal plans and guidance on carbohydrate counting can help manage blood sugar levels.
   - ○ Educational programs on healthy eating can empower individuals to make informed choices.

3. Physical Activity:
   - ○ Encouraging regular exercise tailored to individual capabilities is crucial for managing diabetes.
   - ○ Support systems may include fitness programs, group activities, or personalized exercise plans.

4. Emotional Support:
   - ○ Counseling and support are two things that mental health experts may offer to assist people deal

with the emotional difficulties that come with having diabetes.

- Online forums and support groups can provide a feeling of acceptance and understanding.

5. Education Programs:
- Diabetes education classes covering topics such as blood sugar monitoring, medication management, and lifestyle modifications are beneficial.
- Workshops on stress management and coping strategies can enhance overall well-being.

6. Family and Social Support:
- Involving family members and close friends in the support system ensures a holistic approach to managing diabetes.
- Raising awareness and fostering understanding among friends and family helps create a supportive environment.

7. Technology Integration:
- Utilizing diabetes management apps, wearable devices, and continuous glucose monitors can empower individuals to track and

> manage their condition
> effectively.
- Telehealth services facilitate remote monitoring and consultations.

8. Regular Monitoring:
   - Encourage regular monitoring of blood sugar levels and other relevant health indicators to detect any changes promptly.
   - Implementing a routine for self-monitoring reinforces accountability and proactive management.

9. Financial Support:
   - Assistance programs or insurance coverage for diabetes-related expenses can alleviate financial burdens.
   - Access to affordable medications and supplies is crucial for ongoing management.

10. Community Resources:
    - Connecting individuals with local or online diabetes support groups fosters a sense of community and shared experiences.
    - Access to resources such as educational materials,

workshops, and events enhances diabetes management.

By incorporating these components into a comprehensive support system, individuals with Type 2 diabetes can better navigate the challenges associated with their condition and achieve improved overall health and well-being.

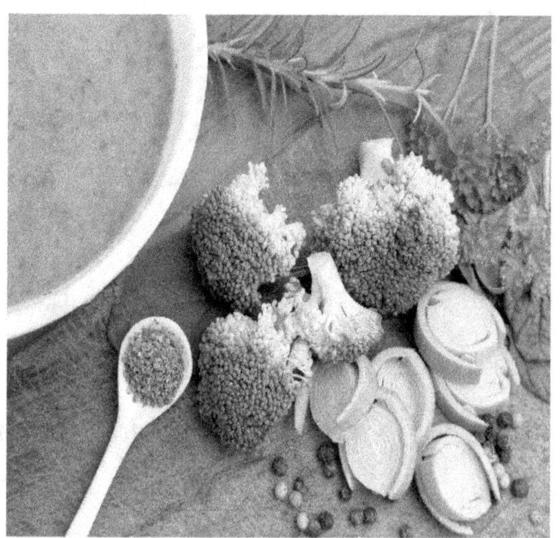

CHAPTER 10
FUTURE TRENDS AND RESEARCH

Future trends and research in Type 2 diabetes are focused on advancing treatment modalities, improving patient outcomes, and addressing the underlying causes of the disease. Precision medicine is gaining prominence, tailoring treatments based on individual genetic, lifestyle, and environmental factors. Personalized therapies aim to enhance efficacy and minimize side effects.

Continuous glucose monitoring (CGM) and wearable technology are anticipated to play a crucial role. Advanced CGM devices offer real-time data, allowing for better management and timely intervention. Integration with artificial intelligence (AI) and machine learning enables predictive modeling, helping individuals and healthcare providers make informed decisions.

The exploration of novel pharmacological agents is ongoing. Researchers are investigating drugs that target specific pathways involved in insulin resistance and glucose regulation. Additionally, there's a growing interest in gut microbiome research, as it is implicated in metabolic health. Modifying the microbiota may become a potential avenue for managing Type 2 diabetes.

Stem cell therapy and regenerative medicine are emerging as exciting areas of study. Researchers are exploring the potential of regenerating insulin-producing beta cells to restore proper glucose control. While this field is in its early stages, it holds promise for future diabetes treatment strategies.

Digital health interventions, including mobile apps and telemedicine, are becoming integral for diabetes management. These tools facilitate remote monitoring, provide educational resources, and enhance communication between patients and healthcare professionals, leading to improved adherence and outcomes.

Community-based interventions and public health initiatives are gaining attention to prevent and manage Type 2 diabetes on a broader scale. These efforts focus on lifestyle modifications, promoting healthy eating, physical activity, and addressing social determinants of health.

Furthermore, vaccine research for preventing Type 2 diabetes is an intriguing avenue. Targeting specific components related to insulin resistance or beta-cell function, vaccines may offer a preventive measure against the development of the disease.

In conclusion, future trends and research in Type 2 diabetes encompass a multidimensional approach, integrating technological advancements, personalized medicine, and innovative therapeutic strategies. As these avenues progress, the hope is to transform diabetes management, ultimately improving the quality of life for individuals affected by this prevalent metabolic disorder.

CHAPTER 11

RECAP OF KEY POINTS

Type 2 diabetes is a chronic condition that affects how the body regulates and uses sugar (glucose) as a fuel. It occurs when the body becomes resistant to insulin, a hormone that helps glucose enter the cells, or when the pancreas does not produce enough insulin. Type 2 diabetes is the most common form of diabetes, affecting about 10% of the U.S. population and 90%-95% of all people with diabetes

Some of the symptoms of type 2 diabetes are increased thirst, frequent urination, fatigue, weight loss, blurred vision, slow-healing wounds, and infections. However, many people with type 2 diabetes do not have any symptoms or may not notice them for a long time. Therefore, it is important to get regular blood tests to check the glucose levels and diagnose the condition early.

The causes of type 2 diabetes are not fully understood, but they may include genetic, environmental, and lifestyle factors. Some of the risk factors for developing type 2 diabetes are obesity, sedentary lifestyle, family history, age, prediabetes, gestational diabetes, and polycystic ovarian syndrome. Type 2 diabetes can also lead to serious complications, such as heart disease, stroke, kidney failure, nerve damage, eye problems, and skin infections.

Type 2 diabetes cannot be cured, but it can be managed with healthy habits, medications, and insulin therapy. The main goals of treatment are to lower the blood sugar levels, prevent or delay the complications, and improve the quality of life. Some of the ways to achieve these goals are eating a balanced diet, exercising regularly, monitoring the glucose levels, taking oral or injectable drugs, and using insulin injections or pumps.

Type 2 diabetes is a serious but manageable condition that requires lifelong care and attention. By following the treatment plan, maintaining a healthy lifestyle, and staying in touch with the health care team, people with type 2 diabetes can live long and healthy lives.

IMPORTANT OF DIABETES EDUCATION

An essential part of managing and caring for diabetes is diabetes education.

It helps people with diabetes learn how to cope with their condition, make healthy lifestyle choices, monitor their blood sugar levels, take their medications, prevent or delay complications, and improve their quality of life. Diabetes education is also known as diabetes self-management education and support (DSMES).

According to the Centers for Disease Control and Prevention (CDC), DSMES services provide people with diabetes with knowledge and tools to manage their health in a way that works for them and their lifestyle. DSMES is guided by national standards and covers seven self-care behaviors: healthy coping, healthy eating, being active, taking medication, monitoring, problem-solving, and reducing risk.

DSMES can benefit people with diabetes in many ways. Research has shown that DSMES can help people improve their blood sugar levels, lower their risk of heart disease and stroke, reduce health care costs, and enhance their well-being.

DSMES can also help people adjust to new situations, such as changes in treatment, health status, or life circumstances.

DSMES services are available in various settings, such as hospitals, clinics, community centers, and online platforms. People with diabetes can access DSMES through referrals from their health care providers or by searching for accredited or recognized programs near them[1]. Some insurance plans, including Medicare, cover DSMES services for eligible people with diabetes.

Diabetes education is not a one-time event, but a lifelong process that requires ongoing support and reinforcement. People with diabetes should seek DSMES services at different times in their diabetes journey, such as at diagnosis, annually, when new complications arise, or when transitioning to new phases of life. By participating in DSMES, people with diabetes can gain the confidence and skills to manage their diabetes effectively and live a healthy and fulfilling life.

CONCLUSION

In conclusion, managing Type 2 diabetes is a multifaceted challenge that requires a holistic approach encompassing lifestyle modifications, medication adherence, and regular monitoring. With advancements in medical research and technology, there is hope for improved treatment options and better outcomes. However, individual responsibility remains crucial in maintaining a healthy lifestyle and minimizing the impact of this chronic condition. Education, awareness, and ongoing support are key elements in empowering individuals to navigate the complexities of Type 2 diabetes and enhance their overall well-being.

www.ingramcontent.com/pod-product-compliance
Lightning Source LLC
Chambersburg PA
CBHW070950250726

48663CB00002B/158